Self-Assessment Colour Review
Dermatology

Ronald Marks

BSc (Hons), DTM&H, FRCP, FRCPath
Emeritus Professor, University of Wales College of Medicine
Cardiff, UK

ЗHING

For full details of all Manson Publishing Ltd titles please write to:
Manson Publishing Ltd, 73 Corringham Road, London NW11 7DL, UK.
Tel: +44(0)20 8905 5150
Fax: +44(0)20 8201 9233
Email: manson@mansonpublishing.com
Website: www.mansonpublishing.com

Commissioning editor: Jill Northcott
Project manager: Paul Bennett
Copyeditor: Joanna Brocklesby and Ruth Maxwell
Design and layout: Cathy Martin
Indexer: Dr Laurence Errington
Colour reproduction: Tenon & Polert Colour Scanning Ltd, Hong Kong
Printed by: New Era Printing Co Ltd, Hong Kong

Preface

Dermatology and ophthalmology are reputedly the two specialties in medicine that have the 'most diseases'. If this is the case, it may be because in only these two specialties, compared to all the others, the disorder is obvious. This makes dermatology a special skill, tending to attract the 'Sherlock Holmes'-type of physician. This kind of individual will, in clinical practice, assiduously look for clues and will experience genuine pleasure when involved in the deductive process. This book should satisfy his/her intellectual lust.

The book has additional other important purposes. It has been recognized since the 'beginning of time' that there is no better way of learning than being tested time and time again. The collection of questions and answers in this book covers most aspects of clinical dermatology and once its content has been mastered the reader will have made an important start to being proficient at sorting out (recognizing) skin disorders.

Ronald Marks

Acknowledgements

I gratefully acknowledge the assistance of Dr Richard Goodwin in assembling the illustrations.

I am also extremely grateful to the Department of Medical Illustration of University Hospital of Wales for taking many of the photographs.

Abbreviations

AA	alopecia areata
CDLE	chronic discoid lupus erythematosus
CDNCH	chondrodermatitis nodularis chronica helicis
DM	dermatomyositis
DSAP	disseminated superficial actinic porokeratosis
EB	epidermolyis bullosa
EBA	epidermolyis bullosa acquisita
EM	erythema multiforme
EMPD	extramammary Paget's disease
EN	erythema nodosum
EPS	elastosis perforans serpiginosa
GA	granuloma annulare
HIV	human immunodeficiency virus
HPV	human papillomavirus
HSP	Henoch–Schönlein purpura
IgG	immunoglobulin G
JPD	juvenile plantar dermatosis
NLD	necrobiosis lipoidica diabeticorum
NME	necrolytic migratory erythema
PASI	psoriasis area severity index
PCT	porphyria cutanea tarda
P–J	Peutz–Jeghers disease
PLE	polymorphic light eruption
PLEVA	pityriasis lichenoides et varioliformis acuta
PRP	pityriasis rubra pilaris
PTM	pretibial myxoedema
PUVA	photochemotherapy with ultraviolet A
SLE	systemic lupus erythematosus
SSGH	senile sebaceous gland hyperplasia
TNF-α	tumour necrosis factor alpha
UV	ultraviolet
UVR	ultraviolet radiation

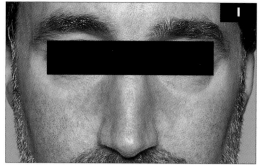

1 A male complains of increasingly severe dandruff and an itchy rash on the face (1). No other area is involved. He is in other respects well and there is no significant history of previous disease. He is prescribed a steroid cream, which provides only temporary relief.
i. What is the most likely diagnosis?
ii. What differential diagnosis should be entertained?
iii. What investigations should be undertaken?

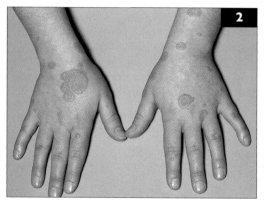

2 A 52-year-old female became ill while on holiday in Kenya. At first there was a faint rash on her trunk. The following day the eruption was very much worse with large deep red blotches all over her skin. She also felt unwell and had a headache and fever. On the third day she was much worse, with the skin showing blistering in places and peeling in others (2). The oral and genital mucosae had also developed erosions.
i. What is the most likely diagnosis? How does it differ from other similar disorders?
ii. What investigations may help in establishing the diagnosis?
iii. Discuss the management.

1 i. The most likely diagnosis is seborrhoeic dermatitis.

ii. The differential diagnosis should include psoriasis, allergic contact dermatitis to a topical application, and atopic dermatitis, although this latter would be unusual occurring for the first time in an adult. Psoriasis is not usually itchy, but certainly can be. Other disorders such as rosacea and lupus erythematosus are seldom itchy.

iii. If there is doubt concerning the clinical diagnosis, it is worth performing a biopsy as although an indeterminate result may not be helpful, a positive result would be conclusive. If a 3 or 4 mm punch biopsy is performed without sutures being inserted, scarring will not be a problem. Patch testing to cosmetics or medicaments will be appropriate if allergic contact dermatitis is suspected. If the patient has severe seborrhoeic dermatitis occurring for the first time, the possibility of human immunodeficiency virus (HIV) disease or other form of immunosuppression should be considered and the appropriate blood tests performed.

2 i. The generalized nature, the severity, and the rapid progression all favour a drug reaction. The picture is more like that of toxic epidermal necolysis than severe erythema multiforme (EM), although there may be overlap in some patients. In EM the mucosal involvement is earlier and more severe and the rash tends to remain in distinct elements rather than becoming generalized. On investigation it was found that she had been taking mefloquine as malaria prophylaxis and this is a rare but recognized cause of toxic epidermal necrolysis in a few subjects.

ii. Skin biopsy showed severe necrotic change in the upper epidermis, with a dense inflammatory cell infiltrate subepidermally and invading the epidermis.

iii. The patient was evacuated by air ambulance back to the UK and was admitted to an intensive care unit. She was treated as though she had severe burns because of the severe dehydration and susceptibility to infection as a result of the extensive damage to the skin barrier. She was also treated with prednisone 60 mg/day. This patient survived, but must be counted as fortunate as there is a mortality rate of approximately 50%.

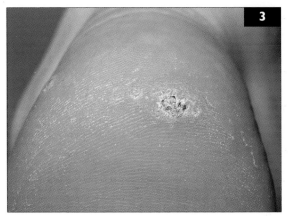

3 i. What is the lesion in 3?
ii. How should it influence its owner's sporting activities?
iii. Discuss the treatments for this condition.

4 A 70-year-old female, who has lived in Florida for the past 30 years, presents with an increasing skin problem on both lower legs. Close examination shows that there are numerous small warty lesions on the fronts of the legs and many brownish macules. She also has many small distinctive round warty patches, which are surmounted by a horny ridge and seem to have an atrophic centre. In addition, there is a crusted plaque (2 × 1.5 cm) in the middle of the left shin.
i. What is the diagnosis?
ii. What other causative agencies have been blamed for the distinctive lesions that she has?
iii. What is the likely diagnosis of the crusted lesion?

5 A patient, who works on a farm, has had a tender red nodule on the dorsum of his right index finger for the last 3 days.
i. What is the most likely diagnosis?
ii. How did he become infected?
iii. Are there any consequences that could be expected?

3 i. The lesion is a plantar wart. Callosities are found at sites of friction, and are not as well marginated. Corns are mostly found on the tarsal arch and do not have tiny black dots on the surface as do plantar warts.
ii. It is customary to recommend that the sufferer avoid swimming because of the risk of spreading wart infection but it is doubtful whether this reduces spread. Plantar warts are quite tender on pressure and some children use this as an excuse to avoid sporting activities, but they should be encouraged to do as much as possible.
iii. In general, treatment is not very effective and is often quite painful. In addition, all plantar warts eventually resolve spontaneously. For these reasons some dermatologists recommend reassurance without active treatment. Active treatments are all destructive and include freezing with liquid nitrogen or solid carbon dioxide (cryotherapy), surgical removal by curettage and cautery, ablation by laser beam, or chemotherapy with keratolytics (high concentrations of salicylic acid) or antimitotic agents, such as podophyllin extracts or bleomycin.

4 i. The diagnosis is almost certainly chronic solar damage with numerous solar keratoses, solar lentigines, and lesions of disseminated superficial actinic porokeratosis (DSAP).
ii. Lesions of porokeratosis have been blamed on immunosuppression, genetic factors, and solar exposure.
iii. The crusted lesion is almost certainly either a squamous cell carcinoma or a basal cell carcinoma – both of which are more frequent in sun-damaged sites and where there are lesions of porokeratosis.

5 i. The most likely diagnosis is orf. This is an infection caused by a DNA virus of the poxvirus group, which spreads to man from sheep and goats.
ii. The hands and fingers are sites commonly involved as the infection is transmitted by contact with affected sites.
iii. The condition usually lasts 10–14 days and heals without scarring. However, in a significant proportion of affected individuals an attack of erythema multiforme follows some 2–4 weeks later.

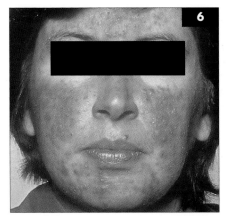

6 A female was 24 years of age when she first noticed that she was blushing much more frequently than she had done previously and that the flushes lasted for longer than they used to. Not only did she blush at minor embarrassments, but she flushed deeply with spicy food and alcoholic drinks. Now, aged 29, she presents because of the persistent redness of her cheeks, chin, and forehead, and the 'pimples' that have appeared in the red areas (6). These seem to come in crops and are sometimes accompanied by pustules.
i. What is the differential diagnosis?
ii. What investigations will help establish a diagnosis?
iii. What are the treatment options for the most likely diagnosis?

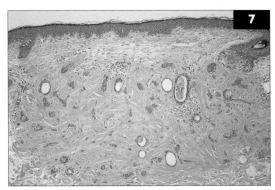

7 i. What condition is presented in this photomicrograph (7)?
ii. What clinical features develop in this condition?
iii. What treatment should be recommended?

6 i. The most likely diagnosis is rosacea, but the differential diagnosis includes seborrhoeic dermatitis, although this disorder is scaly (rosacea is not) and also affects the scalp and facial flexures. In contrast, rosacea mostly affects the facial convexities. The differential diagnosis also includes systemic lupus erythematosus (SLE) and dermatomyositis (DM). The former is a systemic disorder which is accompanied by multiple positive laboratory findings including the presence of anti-DNA antibodies, anaemia, leucopenia, and thrombocytopenia. DM is distinguished by the facial rash having a mauve–lilac hue (heliotrope) and occurring mainly on the upper face as well as the back of the hands. Limb girdle muscular weakness and tenderness accompany the skin disorder. Neither of these conditions causes papules or pustules to appear on affected skin.

ii. A full blood picture, a test for anti-DNA antibodies, and a blood test for muscle enzymes would help exclude SLE and DM. A skin biopsy would distinguish between SLE and rosacea as in the former there is tight 'cuffing' of the small blood vessels with lymphocytes and degenerative changes in the basal epidermal cells. Direct immunofluorescence tests would detect deposits of immunoglobulin G (IgG) and complement component C3 at the dermoepidermal junction in lupus erythematosus.

iii. The treatment of choice for acute rosacea is oral tetracycline. It has been suggested that it is the anti-inflammatory effect rather than any antibacterial action that is responsible for improvement. All the tetracyclines reduce the number of papules and calm the inflammation within 3–4 weeks. A low dose of doxycycline can be administered once or twice daily and is very well tolerated (50 mg twice daily). Oral erythromycin is also effective. Topical metronidazole gel (0.75%) used twice daily is quite effective as is topical azelaic acid cream (20%). Pulsed dye laser treatment has been shown to improve the redness and flushing considerably.

7 i. The condition is the 'naevoid disorder' of sweat gland elements known as syringoma. The histological picture must be carefully distinguished from morphoeic basal cell carcinoma and the rarer condition of desmoplastic trichoepithelioma.

ii. Characteristically small (1–2 mm) pink papules occur on the lower eyelids and on the upper cheeks. In some cases very large numbers of papules also occur over the trunk and limbs. They may do so over relatively short periods of time and the condition is then known as 'eruptive hidradenoma'.

iii. Unfortunately, the only available treatment is the ablation of individual lesions, for example by laser ablation.

8 Severe sunburn affecting the face, upper trunk, and arms is unlikely to occur in northern Europe.
i. Comment on this statement.
ii. Briefly discuss the aetiopathogenesis and pathology of sunburn.
iii. What may be the long-term sequelae of repeated or chronic sunburn?

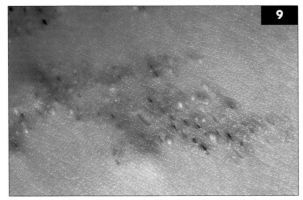

9 A 30-year-old male has been aware of what he called a birth mark on the left side of his abdomen since early childhood (9). In the past few years occasional inflamed spots have developed in the affected area.
i. What is this condition?
ii. Why do inflamed spots develop on the lesion?
iii. Name related naevoid conditions.

8 i. Sunburn can certainly occur in northern Europe depending on the time of year, the length of the exposure, and the vulnerability of the subject. The vulnerability of the subject is primarily a function of the depth of his or her pigmentation.

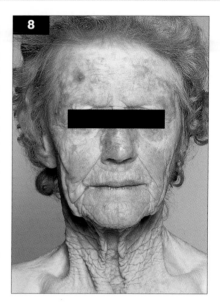

ii. Sunburn is primarily due to a critical dose of solar ultraviolet radiation (UVR) – in particular UVR in the medium waveband (known as UVB) of 190–220 nm band width. The UVB penetrates the epidermis but does not penetrate into the dermis. The damage caused to the epidermal cells results in cell death (sunburn cells), spongiosis, subepidermal blistering, and general inflammatory change. The process is complex, involving activation of the prostaglandin cascade and DNA damage with the formation of thymidine dimers.

iii. Because damage from solar exposure does not cause dermal destruction, scarring and keloid formation do not result. Similarly, permanent alteration in pigmentation does not occur. However, exposure to UVR in the long term causes both melanoma and nonmelanoma skin cancer. The present day epidemic of melanoma and the increase in incidence of basal cell carcinoma, solar keratosis, and squamous cell carcinoma is due mostly to the increased annual dose of UVR. Apart from these important results of 'chronic burning', the altered appearance of exposed skin with its lines and wrinkles and yellowish discolouration, known as solar elastosis, causes considerable cosmetic disability (8).

9 i. This is a comedone naevus, a type of epidermal hamartoma in which there are many follicular canals packed with horny debris (as in ordinary blackheads).

ii. The inflamed spots are analogous to the papules or papulopustules in acne and derive from the comedones.

iii. Related naevoid conditions include warty epidermal naevus, naevus sebaceous, 'organoid naevus'.

10 A 27-year-old male has had attacks of diarrhoea with blood and mucus since the age of 18. He appeared otherwise quite well and seemed to respond to oral sulfasalazine. During a flare-up of his bowel condition last summer he developed some inflamed papules and pustules on the lower legs. These lesions looked like acne, but one spot became larger than the rest and developed into an ulcerated area of 2 cm^2 (10). Despite careful treatment with nonadherent dressings and antibiotics, the open area spread within days to produce an ulcer 4 cm^2 in area. It was shallow and had mauve–blue, slightly undermined edges. Bacteriological swabs grew a mixed bacterial flora; sometimes *Pseudomonas* spp. was recovered, but the lesion did not respond to topical mupirocin.

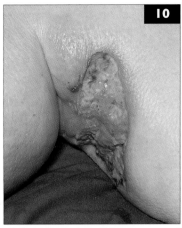

i. What is the differential diagnosis?
ii. Discuss the pathogenesis of the most likely diagnosis.
iii. What treatments are available for the most likely diagnosis?

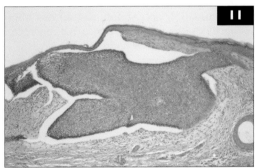

11 A 34-year-old male presents with several darkly pigmented spots on his face, chest, and arms. One of the lesions is removed under local anaesthetic and the pathology is shown in 11. The patient's 12-year-old daughter also has some pigmented spots on her face and chest.
i. What is the diagnosis and why?
ii. Are there any accompanying stigmata or any bone abnormalities that are characteristic of this condition?
iii. Discuss the management of this condition.

13

10 i. The diagnosis is almost certainly pyoderma gangrenosum. This condition occurs in the course of ulcerative colitis and other chronic inflammatory disorders including Crohn's disease and rheumatoid arthritis. It also occurs in para-proteinaemias and leukaemic disorders. In a proportion of cases (perhaps 30%) no underlying cause can be found. It can spread with frightening rapidity, but can also heal quickly. Other ulcerative conditions that should be considered include a form of vasculitis (e.g. polyarteritis nodosa), and a skin infection such as a streptococcal condition or infection with a *Mycobacterium* spp.

ii. Pyoderma gangrenosum is not due to a skin infection. It has been thought to be due to a small vessel vasculitis, but skin biopsies usually do not confirm the presence of this. It is generally assumed that an immunological reaction of some type is involved leading to acute ischaemic ulceration and subsequently infection.

iii. Various treatments have been used and reported as successful including the low-dose tetracyclines minocycline and doxycycline, systemic corticosteroids, dapsone, clofazimine, mycophenolate mofetil, and ciclosporin, the latter drug being the most frequently used. Recently, biological immunomodulators such as infliximab have been used successfully.

11 i. This patient is suffering from the basal cell naevus syndrome (Gorlin's syndrome). The development of multiple pigmented lesions, which turn out to be basal cell carcinomas, in a relatively young individual is quite typical. The development of similar lesions in the patient's daughter is also consistent as the condition is inherited as a Mendelian dominant characteristic.

ii. Minute pits on the palmar skin are a common accompaniment. There may be five or more of these, each less than 1 mm in diameter. Bony abnormalities may occur including cysts in the mandible and bifid ribs. Other abnormalities include frontoparietal bossing of the skull giving a relative macrocephaly and various vertebral abnormalities.

iii. Individual lesions should be removed as they appear. However, excision may become impractical when very large numbers develop and for these patients the use of oral retinoids has proved invaluable. Both isotretinoin and acitretin have been most frequently used and regular administration of one of these greatly reduces the rate of appearance of new lesions. Unfortunately, the regular administration of one of these inevitably causes side-effects (dry lips, loss of hair, dry itchy skin), which makes compliance difficult.

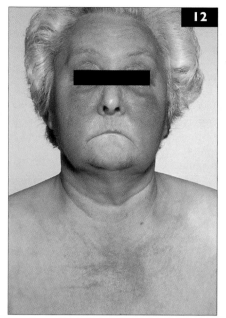

12 A female has developed a rash on her face in the previous 6 weeks and complains that it is gradually worsening (12). She also feels unwell, tired, and weak, and the rash is spreading to other areas of skin. It is particularly difficult to comb her hair and to sit up from the horizontal position. She finds that her shoulders and thighs are quite tender to the touch.
i. What is the diagnosis?
ii. What laboratory tests should be performed to confirm the diagnosis?
iii. What other areas of the skin may be affected?
iv. What diseases may be associated with this disorder?
v. Outline a management strategy for patients affected by this disease.

13 An overweight 64-year-old male presented with a painful, tender red nodule that had developed on the right side of the upper part of the back at the site of a symptomless swelling that he had noted over the past few months. He was prescribed antibiotics, but the condition did not improve. After 3 weeks the centre of the nodule broke down and drained blood-stained yellowish viscid pus.
i. What is the differential diagnosis and what is the most likely diagnosis?
ii. Discuss the pathogenesis and the pathology.
iii. Comment on the management for this condition.

12 i. The diagnosis is dermatomyositis (DM). The lilac–mauve hue to the skin around the eyes and on the upper part of the face is characteristic. It is often described as heliotrope after the flower. Notice the swelling of the periorbital area; this is also quite typical.

ii. Serum muscle enzymes are often much elevated, especially lactic dehydrogenase and aldolase; 24-h urinary creatine is increased. Muscle biopsy will often reveal a characteristic picture with areas of muscle damage, even necrosis and lymphocyte infiltrates. Electromyography will often, but not invariably, show abnormal patterns of electrical activity reflecting the focal nature of the myonecrosis and inflammatory change.

iii. Typically, the paronychial areas of skin are red and swollen and the eponychium develops a ragged distal edge. Reddened patches also appear over the backs of the metacarpals and over the knuckles (known as Gottron's papules). In addition, reddened patches may appear over the elbows and knees. More rarely, areas of inflammation over the trunk and even erythroderma have been recorded.

iv. DM often arises spontaneously for no known reasons, but in some patients the disease seems to signal the presence of a visceral neoplasm. This is especially the case with women over the age of 40 in whom the onset of DM indicates a neoplasm of uterus, ovary, or breast in some 50% of those affected.

v. The aims of management are to relieve the symptoms, prevent the onward progression of the disease, and to determine the presence of any underlying neoplasm. Systemic steroids and immunosuppressive agents in individually designed regimens will halt the progress in the great majority of cases. How far the investigations for underlying neoplastic lesions are carried out is a moot and contentious point. Most would agree that pelvic ultrasound is required in women as well as a thorough investigation of individual symptoms in both sexes.

13 i. The most likely diagnosis is a ruptured epidermoid cyst or a follicular retention cyst. Differential diagnoses include a carbuncle and an acne cyst.

ii. Histologically, the remnants of the cyst wall are usually easily seen. Around the cyst wall there is considerable inflammation with both polymorphs and epithelioid and giant cells. It is believed that the cyst wall ruptures or leaks, stimulating the mixed inflammatory response.

iii. Surgery is usually **not** the answer unless the cyst reforms. Usually the condition subsides within a few weeks without sequelae. It is worthwhile administering a tetracycline such as doxycycline because of the anti-inflammatory effect of this class of antibiotic.

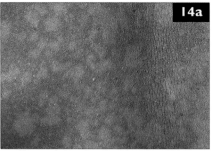
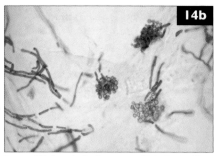

14 A male presents with an increasing number of light pink–brown, slightly scaling macules over the chest, back, and upper arms (**14a**). Skin scrapings stained with periodic acid-Schiff reagent yield the microscopic view seen in **14b**.
i. What is the diagnosis?
ii. What predisposes to this disorder?
iii. Briefly discuss the management.

15 i. What is the Koebner phenomenon?
ii. In what conditions is it seen?
iii. What is the negative Koebner phenomenon?
iv. Briefly state what is known of the cause of the Koebner phenomenon.

16 A 12-year-old female presents with three coin-sized areas of hair loss on the scalp she first noticed 6 months ago. The hair regrew – white at first – and then fell out again.
i. What is the diagnosis and discuss the differential diagnosis?
ii. Are there disease associations of which one should be aware?
iii. Discuss the management.

14 i. The diagnosis is pityriasis versicolor, which is caused by infection with the yeast-like microorganism *Malassezia furfur*, previously known as *Pityrosporon ovale*. The light brown–pink slightly scaling medallions over the trunk are characteristic. The 'spaghetti and meatball' appearance of the spores and pseudohyphae of the yeast microscopically in the skin scrapings is typical.
ii. The yeast is a normal inhabitant of hair follicles and only becomes pathogenic in relatively immunosuppressed states (e.g. after steroid treatments or in Cushing's syndrome) and when personal hygiene is not as meticulous as it could be.
iii. The condition responds to both traditional treatments (e.g. with Whitfield's ointment [benzoic acid and salicylic acid in white soft paraffin]), or treatment with modern topical agents such as one of the imidazoles (e.g. miconazole, clotrimazole, econazole) or a triazole such as ketoconazole. Very extensive disease, stubborn cases, or patients who cannot comply with instructions for topical therapy may require treatment with systemic agents such as oral itraconazole (100 mg daily for 7 days).

15 i. The Koebner phenomenon is the appearance of a pre-exisiting skin disorder at a previously normal site after injury.
ii. The Koebner phenomenon is often seen in psoriasis, but is also observed in lichen planus and discoid lupus erythematosus. It has also been seen in viral warts and molluscum contagiosum.
iii. The negative Koebner phenomenon is the disappearance of a skin disorder at the site of minor injury. It is not infrequently seen in lichen planus.
iv. The complete explanation for the Koebner phenomenon is not known. It appears that the injury has to at least damage upper dermal capillaries.

16 i. The diagnosis is almost certainly alopecia areata (AA). Other conditions causing round discrete areas of hair loss without scarring include ringworm and trichitillomania. When patches of AA are extending, the hairs at the edge show an odd deformity in which the end nearest the scalp is narrowed, so-called 'exclamation mark' hairs. At the start of hair regrowth nonpigmented white hairs appear.
ii. AA is thought to be an autoimmune disease and has been found to be associated with thyroid disease, vitiligo, and rheumatoid arthritis.
iii. Most patients of this age group with limited AA recover completely within a few months and need no treatment. Large stubborn areas may be treated with potent topical corticosteroids, tacrolimus (protopic), or minoxidil 3–5%. Another approach has been to treat the areas with ultraviolet (UV) radiation or psoralen plus UVA treatment. One other form of treatment is to induce an allergic contact dermatitis at the affected site using the potent allergen diphencyprone. A dermatitis develops and after some weeks new hair starts to appear in 60–70% of patients.

17 A 48-year-old male complains that in the previous 3–4 years all his finger and toe nails have changed in colour to a dull yellow, with a greenish hue in places, and have become thicker and very difficult to cut. In addition, the rate of nail growth has slowed enormously and the lateral curvature has increased. On examination (17) there is no eponychium on the nails; the dorsa of the hands, the ankles, and the face appear oedematous. Two of the finger nails have spontaneously been shed some time previously and the abnormal nail has grown back in.

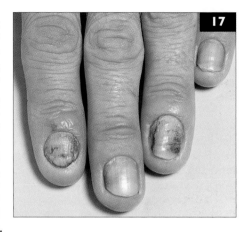

i. What is the name of this disorder, and how common is it?
ii. Describe the medical disorders associated with the condition.
iii. What other nail disorders can cause thickened discoloured nails?

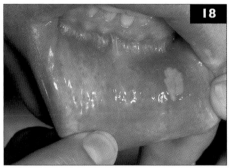

18 A 23-year-old female suffers from recurrent painful mouth ulcers (18); over the previous 3 years she has had four to six attacks of ulcers per year. She also suffers ulcers on the labia and in the vagina and has pain in the wrists and knees with some limitation of movement.

i. What is the most likely diagnosis? What criteria should be satisfied for this diagnosis?
ii. What other disorders are associated with this condition?
iii. What laboratory findings may assist in the diagnosis of this disease?
iv. Briefly discuss the management of this disorder.

17 i. The disorder is known as the yellow nail syndrome. It is extremely uncommon. There are no published statistics but, as an estimate, the average dermatologist may see one such patient every 1 or 2 years.

ii. The condition is associated with pleural effusion, the fluid of which has the qualities of a transudate rather than an exudate and reforms after being drained. The condition is also associated with recurring sinusitis and swelling of the backs of the hands and ankles.

iii. Pachyonychia congenita is responsible for extremely thickened discoloured nails, but this is present from birth in the great majority of cases. There is also hyperkeratosis of the palms and soles; other family members may be affected as it is inherited in a dominant manner. The nails may be thickened and discoloured in psoriasis, but it would be uncommon if there were no accompanying patches of psoriasis on the skin and the nail plates are usually also dystrophic and deformed in this disorder. Ringworm of the nails (tinea unguium) causes irregularly discoloured toe nails with crumbling and irregular nail plates.

18 i. The most likely diagnosis is Behçet's syndrome. The diagnosis is made on clinical criteria – recurrent oral ulceration occurring together with two other major features such as genital ulceration, ocular inflammation, skin lesions, and joint involvement.

ii. Inflammatory ocular disease is an important associated feature. Acute anterior uveitis is typical, but may be accompanied by posterior uveitis and retinal vasculitis. Arthralgia is common and monoarticular arthritis of medium-size joints is not uncommon. Neurological involvement appears to occur quite often with minor symptoms such as headache and disturbances of balance. More serious episodes, such as meningoencephalitis, and brainstem and cerebellar syndromes are much less frequent. The vascular system is also sometimes affected.

iii. The only laboratory finding of any help is 'pathergy'. This is the development of an inflamed, sterile pustule at the site of a minor injury to the skin such as a needle prick.

iv. Topical or systemic corticosteroids may control the ulcers. Oral colchicine has also been found helpful for some patients. For intractable ulceration short courses of thalidomide have been found helpful, but this must be given with care.

19 A girl was born with a large angioma on her leg (**19**). Over some weeks the lesion has enlarged disproportionally and at one stage an erosion appeared, which oozed and bled a little.
i. What is the lesion known as?
ii. What complications can occur?
iii. What treatments are available for such lesions?

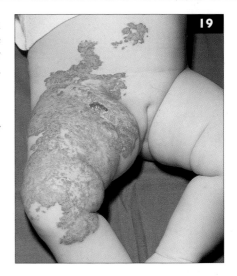

20 i. What is the creature illustrated in **20**? Where does it live? What are the differences between the sexes?
ii. What are the typical features of the disease it causes?
iii. How does one catch this disorder? What is the incubation period?
iv. Discuss the management of this disorder.

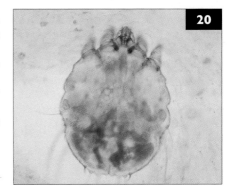

21 A female complains of the recurrent appearance of painful bruises after emotional stress or on occasion after a minor physical injury. Exhaustive routine investigations do not reveal any abnormalities to account for the bleeding.
i. What is the most likely diagnosis and what are the differential diagnoses?
ii. Are there any characteristic accompanying features of the most likely diagnosis?
iii. What is known of the aetiopathogenesis of the most likely diagnosis?

19 i. Such lesions are usually known as 'strawberry naevus' or 'strawberry angioma'.
ii. Erosion, with bleeding and sometimes infection, is common. In large lesions sequestration of platelets can occur causing a bleeding diathesis.
iii. Usually no treatment is required as the lesions tend to reduce in size later and spontaneously involute in childhood. Laser ablation may be tried with smaller lesions. Larger lesions have been treated successfully with intralesional injections of corticosteroids, interferon-gamma, or topical imiquimod.

20 i. This is the scabies mite (*Sarcoptes scabiei*) – the mite that causes human scabies. The mite that causes dog scabies and the mites that cause scabies in other mammals are each slightly different. It burrows and lives in tunnels within the superficial stratum corneum (scabies 'runs'). The female is the larger of the two sexes and the one that burrows into the stratum corneum, causing scabies. The male is much smaller and hardly ever seen.
ii. Scabies is characterized by intense pruritus and the sudden onset of an itching rash with multiple excoriations on a background of eczema and prurigo papules. Lesions are often found on the hands (palms and between the fingers), on the wrists and elbows, around the anterior axillary folds, around the nipples, around the umbilicus, on the buttocks, and on the genitalia – papules on the shaft of the penis and scrotum are typical.
iii. The disease is caught by skin-to-skin contact, so sexual contact is an extremely common means of passing on the infestation. It also spreads rapidly within families and institutions. The incubation period is approximately 4 weeks for the first attack, but may only be a few days in second and subsequent attacks.
iv. The infected individual and all his or her close contacts need to be treated at the same time. After a hot bath the entire skin surface from the neck down is treated with permethrin cream (5%). Another bath after 8–10 h is followed by a further application of the cream and another after 7 days. Other scabecidal agents that are now not often used include benzyl benzoate lotion, gammexane, malathion, crotamiton, and sulphur.

21 i. The most likely diagnosis is the autoerythrocyte sensitization syndrome – also known as the Gardner-Diamond syndrome. Idiopathic thrombocytopenic purpura, anaphylactoid purpura, and factitial purpura are other differential diagnoses that should be considered.
ii. Malaise and fever may accompany the appearance of the ecchymoses. Intracutaneous injection of washed autologous erythrocytes may provoke lesions within 24 h.
iii. Very little is known of the aetiopathogenesis other than attacks occur in middle-aged females.

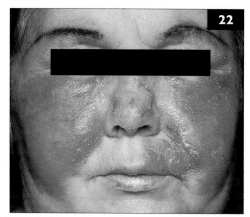

22 An 80-year-old female has enjoyed excellent health until the sudden onset of a tender bright red rash on the central parts of the face. It has a 'bat's wing' distribution affecting both cheeks and the skin of the bridge of the nose (22). She has a pyrexia and is extremely unwell. Close examination shows that the edge of the affected area of skin is raised and oedematous and markedly haemorrhagic in places.

i. What is she suffering from and what are the differential diagnoses?

ii. What is the cause of the most likely diagnosis?

iii. How can the condition be treated and what is the prognosis?

23 i. List the main aetiological factors in male pattern alopecia.

ii. Does this condition occur in women? If so discuss the main differential diagnoses.

iii. Briefly discuss the management options for male pattern alopecia in a man of 40 who is very concerned over his appearance.

22 i. This patient has erysipelas. The sudden onset of a tender rash with a well-defined border and an accompanying pyrexial illness are all typical of this condition. Rosacea and systemic lupus erythematosus (SLE) should be considered in the differential diagnosis. Rosacea affects mostly the convex facial surfaces; there is no distinct edge to the rash as well as there being no systemic component. In SLE other areas of skin are often affected and additional organ systems may be involved such as the renal system or the heart.

ii. The cause of erysipelas is infection with beta-haemolytic *Streptococcus*, although it is often difficult to recover the microorganism from swabs or the affected tissues, and only very small numbers can be identified in tissue sections of biopsies of the rash. It has been suggested that the reason for this is that the condition results from hypersensitivity to the beta-haemolytic *Streptococcus* rather than any direct toxic effects of the microorganism.

iii. Erysipelas rapidly responds to penicillin-type antibiotics. After administration of the antibiotic by the intramuscular or intravenous route the temperature should fall and the condition rapidly resolve.

23 i. The main aetiological factors include the inheritance of susceptibility genes, the presence of androgens, and increasing age.

ii. The condition certainly does occur in women, but is not as common and is rarely as severe as in men. There are also some minor clinical differences in that bitemporal recession is seen less commonly in women. The condition must be distinguished from generalized diffuse hair loss seen in women, traction alopecia in which hair loss occurs at certain sites because of mechanical traction, and hair loss due to a type of alopecia areata.

iii. The decision as to whether to offer treatment will depend on the cosmetic issues and wishes of the patient, as well as financial considerations and the local availability of surgical treatments. Topical minoxidil (5%) does stimulate hair growth in up to one-third of patients who use it, but only for so long as treatment is continued. Topical anti-androgens are not suitable for men as the anti-androgen may be absorbed and undesirable feminizing effects then occur systemically. Hair transplants provide a long-term answer for some subjects who have good hair growth at the scalp margins, are prepared for the discomfort and inconvenience, and can afford the procedure. The procedure requires considerable skill and experience.

24 A female presents with a polycyclic erythematous rash on the thighs and lower abdomen that has been present for the past 2 months, extending in area slightly in this period (**24a**). She had the condition once previously about 3 years ago and she thinks that it disappeared spontaneously after about 6 months.

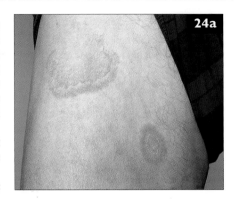

i. What is this condition? What is it usually misdiagnosed as by those clinicians unaware of the condition?

ii. Briefly describe the characteristic histopathological changes.

iii. Name some other similar conditions.

25 **i.** Describe the typical clinical appearance of lichen sclerosus et atrophicus.

ii. Is there a similar disorder affecting men?

iii. What kind of disorder is it often thought to be and are there any other similar conditions?

26 A male presents with a palmar rash (**26**) that has troubled him remittently for the past 2 years. It is worse on the right and, when troublesome, the affected skin fissures and is painful. No other parts of the body are affected.

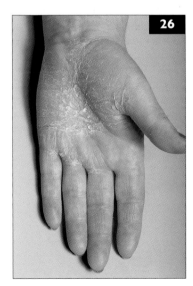

i. What is the differential diagnosis? What is the most likely diagnosis?

ii. What investigations would it be worthwhile doing on this patient?

iii. Indicate the main points to consider when managing this condition.

24 i. This disorder is erythema annulare centrifugum and is usually mistaken for tinea corporis because of the ring-like appearance of the rash.

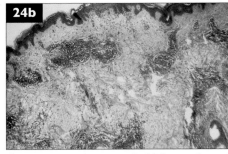

ii. Typically, there is a moderately dense infiltrate of lymphocytes quite closely arranged around the small blood vessels in the upper and mid dermis (24b).

iii. Other similar disorders include erythema gyratum repens (which consists of concentric polycyclic figures and is a sign of visceral neoplasia) and erythema multiforme (which is an acute self-limiting disorder that is often bullous and may affect the mucosae).

25 i. Typically, itchy white atrophic areas appear over the labia and perianally. In a few patients similar areas occur on the trunk ('white spot disease').

ii. The condition of balanitis xerotica obliterans affecting the preputial skin is thought to be the equivalent in men.

iii. Lichen sclerosus is thought to belong to the autoimmune group of disorders. Morphoea may be related as there are some features of the two conditions that overlap.

26 i. The differential diagnoses include chronic hand eczema, psoriasis, ringworm (tinea manuum), tylosis, and lichen planus. The lack of silvery scaling in the crease lines, and the lack of a history of familial involvement or being affected much earlier in life tend to rule out tylosis or psoriasis. The lack of a mauve background hue and an absence of mucosal involvement make lichen planus unlikely. Chronic hand eczema is the most likely diagnosis.

ii. The most appropriate investigations are mycological examination of skin scrapings and patch testing to determine the presence of allergic contact hypersensitivities. A skin biopsy might distinguish psoriasis and lichen planus, but is unlikely to be of much assistance.

iii. Protection of the hands against environmental damage with gloves and barrier creams, the use of bland emollients, and the use of moderately potent topical corticosteroids are the mainstays of treatment.

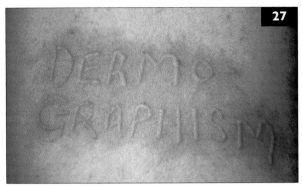

27 i. Are dermographism (27) and pressure urticaria essentially the same?
ii. How may dermographism be treated?
iii. What is white dermographism?

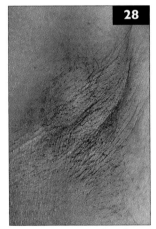

28 A 23-year-old female presents because the skin in her axillae and groins is becoming darker and seems to be thicker and more 'velvety' than normal (28). She has developed many small warty papillomata and skin tags round the axillae and groin area and at the sides of the neck. Her palmar skin seems thicker than previously and velvety. The patient is also considerably overweight, but appears in good health otherwise.
i. What is the differential diagnosis?
ii. What are the main disorders associated with the most likely diagnosis?
iii. Outline the management of the most likely cause of the problem.

27 i. Dermographism and pressure urticaria are quite different. Dermographism (skin writing) is the production of an urticarial weal under a pressure point moving across the skin. It appears within 30 s or so and lasts a few minutes. Pressure urticaria is uncommon and results from strong sustained pressure. It affects an area rather than a line under a moving stylus and lasts for an hour or so.
ii. For the most part dermographism does not need treatment as it is short lived and generally causes trivial discomfort. Antihistamines can prevent or at least diminish the appearance of dermographic weals.
iii. White dermographism is analogous to common dermographism, but the weals that are induced are white. The phenomenon appears to be specific to atopic subjects and may be analogous to 'paradoxical vasoconstriction' seen after intracutaneous injection of acetylcholine analogues. It is unclear whether it is restricted to areas of skin affected by atopic dermatitis or if it also occurs on normal-appearing skin.

28 i. The most likely diagnosis is acanthosis nigricans. As the patient is overweight and appears otherwise quite well the condition is in all probability the variant known as pseudoacanthosis nigricans. The velvety thickening of the skin and the presence of numerous papillomata are typical of all types of acanthosis nigricans. Other possible causes of the increased pigmentation of the flexural areas include Addison's disease, Nelson's syndrome, and pigmentation from drugs. In none of these causes of pigmentation is the flexural accentuation quite so marked or is there an eruption of numerous seborrhoeic wart-like papillomata or thickening of the palmar skin.
ii. Acanthosis nigricans may be provoked by, or be associated with, many systemic disorders. In general terms it may be thought of as commonly associated with obesity, rarely with an underlying neoplastic disorder or, even more rarely, with an endocrine disease or a rare congenital syndrome. The neoplastic disorders are mainly gastrointestinal adenocarcinomata.
iii. The main issue in management is investigation to determine whether there is an underlying cause for the condition. Removal of some of the skin tags and seborrhoeic warts by electrocautery may provide some cosmetic relief.

29 A 27-year-old female has a red patch on her scalp that has become bald in the previous 4 months (29a). She also has a thick red patch about 1.5 cm in diameter on her forehead that seems to be enlarging and has not disappeared in the past 8 weeks.

i. What is the differential diagnosis?

ii. What other physical signs might help in the clinical diagnosis?

iii. Are there any investigations that would help establish the diagnosis?

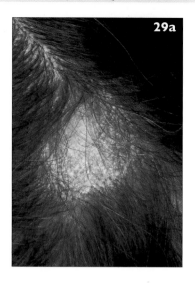

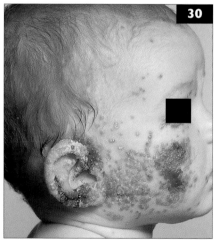

30 A 10-month-old girl is very unwell. The rash she has had since the age of 3 months has suddenly became worse with fever, much inflammation, crusting, and oozing (30).

i. What is the diagnosis?

ii. What is the prognosis? How could this problem be prevented?

iii. Briefly describe the management of this condition.

29 i. The most likely diagnosis is that of chronic discoid lupus erythematosus (CDLE) – the persistence and loss of hair are much in favour of this diagnosis. Bowen's disease and solar keratosis can both be the cause of persistent red patches, but not in the scalp and not usually in a female aged 27 years (>50 years is more likely). Psoriasis, eczema, and ringworm all cause red patches, but their

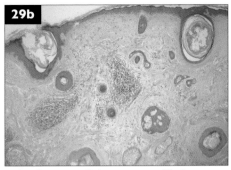

29b

evolution and the lack of other lesions make these conditions very unlikely.

ii. CDLE patches are often slightly scaly and may have horny plugs in the follicle mouths (known as 'tin tack' scales). The lesions are well-defined but irregular in outline and in long-lasting lesions may show scarring and/or pigmentary abnormalities.

iii. The most helpful diagnostic test is skin biopsy. The characteristic picture of perivascular cuffing with lymphocytes in the upper dermis is typical, as are irregular epidermal thickening and hyperkeratosis. In addition, the basal cell layers show degenerative change (29b). Direct immunofluorescence tests on the skin biopsy specimen will reveal immunoglobulin G (IgG) and complement component C3 at the dermoepidermal junction.

30 i. The diagnosis is almost certainly disseminated herpes simplex in a child with atopic dermatitis. This complication of atopic dermatitis is uncommon but not rare. When vaccination against smallpox was a universal public health measure, disseminated vaccinia was occasionally seen in children with atopic dermatitis, and disseminated herpes simplex is a similar but somewhat milder disorder.

ii. Most patients recover completely, although they may be very unwell for a week or thereabouts. The disorder can be prevented by preventing children with atopic dermatitis from coming into contact with individuals with cold sores.

iii. Oozing and crusted areas need to be gently bathed with saline. Aciclovir should be given as early as possible orally. It can also be administered intravenously. Famciclovir is a similar drug that can be used. Some clinicians would also favour giving prophylactic antibiotics at the same time. The underlying eczema needs to be treated with corticosteroids of sufficient strength to suppress the inflammation.

31 i. What is the differential diagnosis of the toe nail problem in 31,
and what is the most likely diagnosis?
ii. What clinical features and what
investigations could help differentiate the conditions?
iii. What treatment should be
recommended for the most likely
diagnosis?

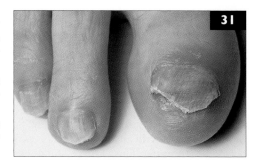

32 A normally healthy 12-year-old
male suddenly developed a widespread papular rash, particularly
marked on his lower legs (32). He
also had considerable pain in his
knees, ankles, wrists, and elbows.
The rash rapidly spread over the
next few days and had a crimson–
purplish colour. Three days later he
has started to complain of colicky
abdominal pain.

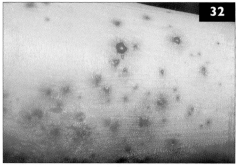

i. What is the diagnosis? Comment on the signs and symptoms.
ii. Describe the pathology of this disorder.
iii. Summarize the management and prognosis of this disorder.

33 i. What is the disorder illustrated
in 33?
ii. What clinical features are typical
of this disease?
iii. Outline its management.

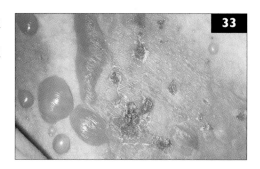

31 i. The two common conditions that need to be distinguished are ringworm of the nails (tinea unguium) and psoriasis of the nails. The involvement of the whole nail plate with thickening and yellow/green/black discolouration tends to favour ringworm but the two conditions are notoriously difficult to distinguish. The most likely diagnosis in this instance is tinea unguium.
ii. A family history of psoriasis, coexistent psoriasis of the skin, and a history of spontaneous improvement and subsequent relapse favour psoriasis. Direct microscopy and culture should always be performed and should settle any doubts.
iii. Treatment is with antifungal agents such as oral terbinafine 250 mg daily for a period of 3 months. This is successful in most patients.

32 i. The diagnosis is that of allergic vasculitis (Henoch–Schönlein purpura; HSP). The purplish papular rash does not fade when pressed with a glass slide because it is purpuric – blood has extravasated into the tissues. The joint pain is due to an allergic synovitis and the abdominal pain is the result of areas of oedema of the gut mucosa and partial intussusseption.
ii. The underlying cause of HSP is that of a small vessel allergic vasculitis characterized by patchy endothelial swelling and even fibrinoid necrosis. Around the sites of endothelial damage there is an inflammatory cell infiltrate composed of polymorphonuclear leucocytes, eosinophils, and fragments of polymorph nuclei ('nuclear dust') – a process known as leucocytoclasis. Some days later in the process lymphocytes replace the polymorphs.
iii. Renal involvement is not uncommon and is the main determinant for prognosis. Without the nephritis HSP rapidly settles without sequelae. Systemic steroids may be needed to improve the arthritis and attacks of abdominal pain.

33 i. The condition illustrated in the photomicrograph is dermatitis herpetiformis.
ii. Intense burning pruritus is highly characteristic. The sites involved are the knees, elbows, buttocks, and scalp, and typically the lesions are urticarial or erythematous patches on which occur clusters of vesicles or small bullae. Diagnosis should be confirmed by biopsy and immunofluorescence examination. Typically, there are subepidermal collections of polymorphs, polymorph debris (or dust), and eosinophils. Direct immunofluorescence testing will reveal immunoglobulin A (IgA) deposition at the papillary tips.
iii. Topical agents will not relieve the severe pruritus. Oral dapsone is the most effective agent – after an adequate dose (50–150 mg) the itching abates within 36 h (usually less). A gluten-free diet improves the well-being of patients with dermatitis herpetiformis, even if the jejunal mucosal abnormality of partial villous atrophy has not been demonstrated. After some months on such a diet the rash improves and the need for dapsone lessens or even disappears.

34 A 28-year-old male presents with a rash over his chest (34a) and back. Every summer the rash becomes more florid, crusted, and exudative. Areas on his face, neck, and scalp also become involved. Apparently his father was similarly affected.
i. What is the diagnosis and how can it be confirmed?
ii. Discuss accompanying physical signs and associations.
iii. Outline the treatment.

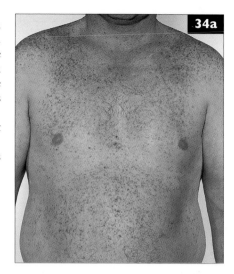

35 A 23-year-old female is very upset by the irregular areas on her lower legs (35).
i. What are the areas?
ii. What investigations should be done?
iii. What is the prognosis?

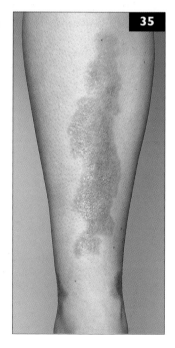

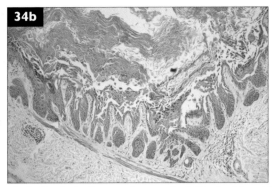

34 i. The diagnosis is Darier's disease (keratosis follicularis), which can be confirmed by biopsy. The histological picture is characterized by suprabasilar clefting and the formation of 'villi' on the basal layer as well as 'partial acantholysis' (34b). In addition, rounded 'corps ronds' and smaller denser 'grains' are found in the upper epidermis amongst the parakeratotic debris.
ii. Tiny pits occur on palmar skin in more than half of patients with Darier's disease. Vertical striations in nail plates leading to 'nicks' in the nail free edge are found in 25–30% of patients. In some families with Darier's disease there is linkage with a psychiatric (schizo-affective) complaint.
iii. The treatment depends on the extent and the severity of the condition. When the condition affects small areas and is not severe, it may be treated with topical (or systemic) antibiotics, topical retinoids and topical steroids, and symptomatic measures alone. When the condition is more extensive and disabling, systemic retinoid drugs do provide significant relief while they are being given (such as acitretin 0.5–1.0 mg/kg daily).

35 i. Persistent pink–yellow irregular plaques showing areas of atrophy over the shins are very likely to be necrobiosis lipoidica diabeticorum (NLD). There are no other conditions that look quite like this, although pretibial myxoedema, which may also occur over the shins, may confuse the inexperienced. It is said that patients with NLD either have, or will have, diabetes mellitus within 5 years, or have a first-degree relative who has, or will have, diabetes mellitus.
ii. Skin biopsy should be performed to confirm the diagnosis. Blood sugar tests and other blood investigations should be performed to characterize the diabetic status.
iii. Currently, there is no treatment that can be employed either topically to the skin disorder itself or systemically for the diabetes that influences NLD. The condition persists for long periods, but becomes less prominent over several months or years leaving a scarred area.

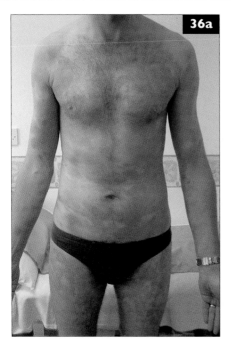

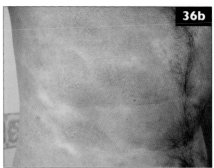

36 A patient presents with a rash that has developed gradually over a 7-year period. It is slightly itchy and unresponsive to multiple topical treatments. The individual elements are rounded or oval and vary in size from 2 to 5 cm. They are red and scaly and some are slightly raised (36a, b).
i. What is the differential diagnosis?
ii. How was the diagnosis confirmed?
iii. Discuss the management.

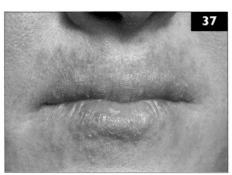

37 A 7-year-old male presents with a rash around his mouth (37) that has been present for the past 3 months. Nothing seems to help.
i. What is the diagnosis?
ii. What is the treatment and prognosis?
iii. List at least three other disorders with an analogous aetiopathogenesis.

36 i. A diagnosis of mycosis fungoides (cutaneous T-cell lymphoma) must be seriously considered. A slowly progressive rash over several years without remissions and unresponsive to treatment is unlikely to be psoriasis or eczema. Ringworm is generally much less extensive and more rapidly progressive.

ii. The diagnosis has to be confirmed histologically. The presence of large abnormal lymphocytes in the subepidermal zone or actually within the epidermis is characteristic. Lymphocytes tend to collect in microabscesses within the epidermis (Pautrier microabscesses). Immunocytochemical tests for 'clonality' should also be performed.

iii. The management depends on the stage of the disease. In the very early stages symptoms may be improved by the use of emollients and moderately potent or potent topical corticosteroids. When the condition is slightly further advanced and the lesions are just palpable, treatment by phototherapy is frequently sufficient to control the disease. Photochemotherapy with ultraviolet A (PUVA) using 8-methoxypsoralen as an ultraviolet-sensitizing agent is employed. Adding oral aromatic retinoids (e.g. acitretin) appears to enhance the efficacy of the PUVA. When the condition is further advanced a variety of treatments have been tried, including electron beam therapy. These are mainly useful to control local symptoms or help produce a temporary remission, but none appears to extend the life of the patient or influence the course of the disease. Various chemotherapy regimens have been tried without much benefit.

37 i. This condition is known as lip-licking cheilitis and is due to the habit of licking the lips frequently. It is thought that the constant wetting and drying causes a dermatitic reaction. It is often misdiagnosed as perioral dermatitis. The micropapular nature and the distribution around the nasolabial grooves serves to distinguish perioral dermatitis.

ii. Discussion and persuasion are usually sufficient to stop the habit, and the use of an unpleasant tasting emollient helps! This is usually a transient disorder.

iii. Other conditions caused by the patient's own actions (conscious, semi- or unconscious) include acne excoriée, dermatitis artefacta, and nodular prurigo.

38 A male presents with spots and small blisters on his penis, which are sore and inhibit any sexual activity. It is the first time that he has had anything like this on his penis. The spots have been present for the previous 4 days.
i. What is the most likely diagnosis?
ii. How may the diagnosis be confirmed?
iii. Outline the management of this problem.

39 The lesion in **39a** appeared on the forearm a few weeks ago.
i. What is the most likely diagnosis and what is the main differential diagnosis?
ii. Figure **39b** shows the pathological picture. What are the main diagnostic features?
iii. What is the management of the most likely diagnosis?

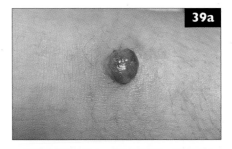

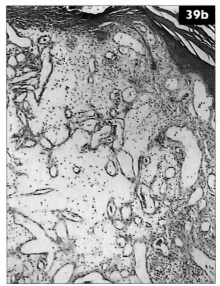

38 i. The most likely diagnosis is herpes simplex infection. Genital herpes infection is usually caused by herpes simplex type 2 virus, but the type 1 virus can also be responsible. Interestingly, labial herpes can only be caused by the type 1 virus. In the male the grouped vesicles or erosions are usually on the prepuce or on the glans penis. In women the labia, cervix, or vagina can be affected. The primary infection is usually more severe than subsequent attacks and may last up to 10 days. Secondary attacks often occur three to five times per year and last 4–6 days. The erosions and vesicles are small and grouped and should not be confused with other causes of genital ulceration including lesions of Behçet's disease, syphilis, and chancroid.

ii. The diagnosis should be confirmed by identification of the virus by culture or by polymerase chain reaction after taking a swab. These techniques have both high sensitivity and high specificity. Serological tests are also available but have less specificity than viral identification techniques. Tzanck smears may assist if giant cells are seen but the test has low sensitivity and specificity.

iii. Infected individuals should be counselled concerning their infectivity. Simple cleansing analgesic gels and antimicrobial measures are usually sufficient, as there are no curative treatments. Current drugs may reduce the severity and length of the disease and may lengthen the periods of remission. These drugs include aciclovir, famciclovir and valaciclovir. Aciclovir may be taken orally and used topically. One dosage regimen is 400 mg three times a day, orally.

39 i. The most likely diagnosis is pyogenic granuloma, but it should be remembered that amelanotic melanoma may be almost indistinguishable clinically.

ii. There are large numbers of thin-walled immature capillaries set in a homogeneous background matrix that also contains large numbers of inflammatory cells.

iii. These lesions should be removed by curettage and cautery and always sent for histological examination.

40 A qualified children's nurse presents with painful and tender red nodules on the extensor surfaces of her lower legs which developed over a weekend.
i. What is the most likely diagnosis and what other disorders have to be considered?
ii. What other clinical features may accompany the most likely diagnosis?
iii. What are the possible aetiologies of the most likely diagnosis?

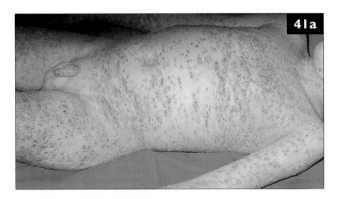

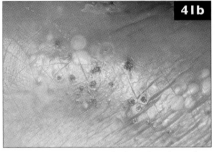
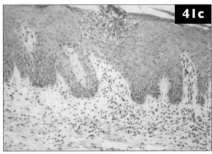

41 A 15-year-old male has developed a generalized pustular eruption (41a, b) over the previous week. There is no previous history or family history of skin disorder. The pustular rash seems to come in waves and the patient develops 'spikes' of pyrexia coincident with the appearance of the pustules. At the same time he complains of feeling unwell and develops pain in the knees, ankles, and elbows. A full blood picture shows the presence of a high polymorphonuclear leucocytosis of $17 \times 10^9/L$. A biopsy is performed and the section is illustrated in 41c.
i. What is the differential diagnosis?
ii. Comment on the pathological changes in 41c.
iii. Discuss the management of this patient.

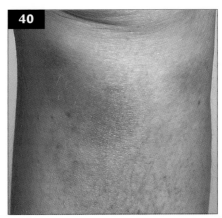

40 i. The most likely diagnosis is erythema nodosum (EN). Other disorders such as nodular vasculitis, polyarteritis nodosa, and erythema induratum may cause painful red nodules but in none of these are the nodules large, tender, and mainly on the shins (40). If there is doubt, a biopsy distinguishes EN because EN is essentially a panniculitis with vasculitic involvement of the interlobular septa and marked extravasation of blood in the tissues.

ii. The nodules are exquisitely tender and leave a bruise when the lesions fade. EN is often accompanied by an arthropathy, with painful ankles and sometimes knees.

iii. Pulmanary tuberculosis, sarcoidosis, persistent streptococcal infection, and administration of some sulfa drugs account for some 50% of cases. No agent can be found responsible in the rest.

41 i. The most likely diagnosis is generalized pustular psoriasis (Von Zumbusch's disease). Other conditions that need to be considered include generalized pustular drug reaction, subcorneal pustulosis (Sneddon Wilkinson disease), generalized herpes simplex (in someone with widespread atopic dermatitis), and (in a pregnant woman) impetigo herpetiformis.

ii. The epidermis is thickened and is permeated by polymorphonuclear leucocytes, which have aggregated to form a small abscess.

iii. Such patients are usually dehydrated, pyrexial, and feel very unwell. Because of these considerations and the skilled nursing attention that their skin condition needs, they frequently require inpatient treatment until the acute episode has passed. Topical treatments are not of any help to these patients. They require systemic immunosuppressive agents such as methotrexate or ciclosporin. The newer 'biological agents' (e.g. etanercept or infliximab) may also be needed.

42 A patient presents with lesions on the palms of the hands. First the right hand developed yellowish and yellow–brown pustules over the palm and then after 6 weeks the left hand began to develop similar lesions (42).
i. What is the most likely diagnosis?
ii. Describe the natural history of this disorder.
iii. What is the pathology of this condition and what is known of the aetiopathogenesis?

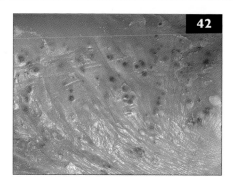

43 A 54-year-old female advertising executive is concerned about her facial appearance (43).
i. What facial features might concern her and how were they caused?
ii. What non-surgical treatments can be recommended to improve her appearance?
iii. What cosmetic surgical interventions are sometimes recommended?

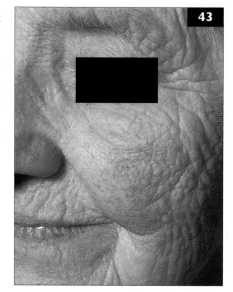

44 A male presents with 'smelly feet'. On examination the horny layers of the soles of the feet are pale, sodden, and fissured or pitted in places.
i. What is the diagnosis?
ii. What is the cause?
iii. What is the treatment for this condition?

42 i. Pustular psoriasis of the palms and soles.
ii. The condition is episodic and chronic, each episode lasting a few weeks to months over several years.
iii. The typical pathological changes are the presence of minute collections of polymorphonuclear leucocytes within a slightly thickened epidermis (micro-abscesses). Little is known of the aetiopathogenesis. There does not appear to be a heritable element and it is uncommon for it to coexist with ordinary plaque-type psoriasis. One curious finding which is as yet unexplained, is the very strong association with cigarette smoking.

43 i. The main facial features that she identifies with ageing are the fine lines at the corners of the eyes (crow's feet), the fine lines around her lips, some accentuation of the nasolobial grooves, obvious crease lines on the forehead, and slight yellowing of the skin surface. Most of these changes have been caused by ultraviolet radiation (UVR) from long-term solar exposure causing the degenerative change in the dermis known as solar elastosis. The forehead creases and nasolabial folds appear to be due to intrinsic ageing.
ii. Reduction in sun exposure will very gradually (over many months) allow repair of the dermis. Use of topical retinoids (such as tretinoin) stimulates dermal repair and produces clinical improvement, but takes several months and is not tolerated by all patients. Chemical peeling using glycolic or trichloracetic acid preparations also stimulates dermal repair. The crease lines on the forehead and the nasolabial folds can be reduced by intracutaneous injection of botulinum toxin, which paralyses the facial muscles so that the skin flattens as the muscles relax; this effect remains for 3–5 months. Intracutaneous injection of inert dermal 'fillers' (often based on hyaluronic acid) can also be used to reduce the contours.
iii. There are numerous lifts, nips, and tucks that experienced skin surgeons use to reduce facial lines and wrinkles.

44 i. The diagnosis is pitted keratolysis (the older term was keratoma plantare sulcatum). It is mainly seen in young men who sweat excessively.
ii. There is some uncertainty as to the bacteriological cause – *Micrococcus sedentarius* or a *Corynebacterium* may be involved.
iii. The condition should be treated with antimicrobial agents, such as the imidazoles or topical erythromycin, and by reducing the sweating with 10% formalin solution, aluminium hexachlorhydrate, or some other measure.

45 A 37-year-old female presents with a 'summer itch', which she started to suffer from at the age of 20 and has gradually worsened each year. The rash affects mainly the arms (45) but sometimes the upper chest, neck, or face are also involved. The rash is erythematous and papular, although sometimes it is more scaly. It is very itchy and causes much discomfort. The rash

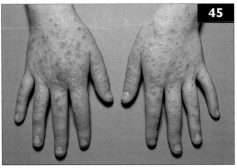

subsides in early autumn and does not trouble the patient again until the following spring.
i. Discuss the differential diagnosis.
ii. What is known about the cause of the most likely diagnosis?
iii. Discuss the management of the most likely diagnosis.

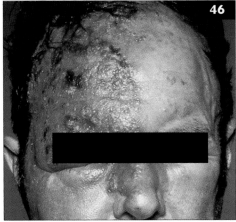

46 The patient in 46 complained of quite severe pain in the region some 3–4 days before the rash appeared. He said that he thought he had been in contact with his nephew, who had chicken pox at the time, and he thought that this contact might have been the cause.
i. What is the diagnosis?
ii. Was he right about his nephew being the cause?
iii. Outline the management.

45 i. The rash develops in the summer and on light-exposed areas of skin, so it is likely to be a photodermatosis. The appearance of the rash and its itchiness are in favour of the diagnosis of polymorphic light eruption (PLE). Alternative diagnoses that ought to be considered include atopic dermatitis, which is sometimes worsened by sun exposure, and photoallergic contact dermatitis (e.g. photoallergy to a constituent of a sunscreen).

ii. Very little is known about the cause of PLE other than a broad range of wavelengths seem to be able to precipitate the condition.

iii. Management may be along two tracks. The first is rigorous protection against sun exposure including sunscreens that have good protection in the ultraviolet A (UVA) range. The second is 'conditioning' of the skin by exposure to increasing doses of ultraviolet radiation starting a few weeks before the condition usually begins. This is quite effective, but must be repeated every year. Any 'breakthrough' rash can be treated by moderate-potency topical corticosteroids.

46 i. The diagnosis is ophthalmic zoster (herpes zoster ophthalmicus). Note that the affected area is swollen and quite well delineated. The disorder is restricted to the distribution of the ophthalmic branch of the trigeminal nerve, apart from there being a few scattered vesiculopustules over the trunk and limbs (which look like chicken pox lesions).

ii. The patient was incorrect about the cause. Patients with zoster might cause varicella (chicken pox) in individuals who have not had chicken pox previously, but they do not cause zoster in contacts. Herpes zoster is not 'caught' from patients with varicella.

iii. The management is first directed at relieving the pain, which may be considerable, using conventional analgesics or, if necessary, opioid drugs; any secondary infection is treated with topical antibiotics. Bathing and gentle removal of crusts will also help. Treatment with systemic aciclovir, famciclovir, or valaciclovir by intravenous infusion or orally may shorten the disease and reduce the severity if started within the first few days of the eruption. An early ophthalmological consultation is also very important to reduce potential damage to the eye.

47 A male presents with a large brown mole on his back (**47a**). It has grown considerably in size in the previous 3 months and has bled.
i. What is the differential diagnosis?
ii. What clinical signs would assist in reaching a clinical diagnosis?
iii. Figure **47b** shows a photomicrograph of a section of the lesion. What are the diagnosis and prognosis?

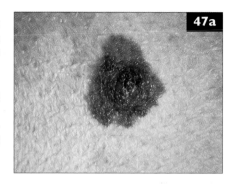

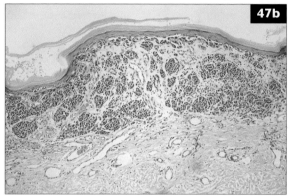

48 A female with a new baby and suffering postnatal depression is experiencing increased hair loss, which has made her even more anxious and tense. The hair loss is diffuse and the hair shafts that are shed seem to have small bulbous ends.
i. What is the most likely cause of the hair loss?
ii. Are there any other causes apart from parturition?
iii. How should the condition be managed?

49 A 78-year-old female presents with painful hard areas on her feet that are making walking difficult. She has had these for 3 years and they are getting worse.
i. What could these areas be?
ii. What is the cause of these lesions?
iii. Briefly discuss the management of these lesions.

47 i. The differential diagnosis includes seborrhoeic wart, malignant melanoma, pigmented basal cell carcinoma, and dermatofibroma.

ii. 'Wartiness', eveness of pigmentation, and the presence of several other similar lesions favours seborrhoeic wart; irregularity of pigmentation and irregularity of border favour a diagnosis of malignant melanoma; a pearlescent appearance overall favours basal cell carcinoma; firmness to palpation favours dermatofibroma.

iii. The histological diagnosis is superficial spreading malignant melanoma. If such an early lesion were completely excised with adequate margins, a 5-year survival rate of 98% is to be expected.

48 i. This condition, which occurs some 3 months after parturition, is known as telogen defluvium. Even in severe cases only 20–30% of the scalp hair is shed. It is due to a proportion of the follicles suddenly being thrown into telogen by the trauma of parturition. Plucking a few strands of hair will reveal a greater proportion with a telogen bulb at the end.

ii. A severe accident, sudden blood loss, or a severe acute infection can also be the cause of telogen defluvium.

iii. Complete recovery always occurs with the normal amount of hair being restored within a few weeks.

49 i. Any localized hyperkeratotic lesion on the sole of the foot may be painful and tender, but the most common cause in this age group is callosity, followed by corns (clavus), and, much less frequently in this age group, by plantar warts. Callosities are mostly found over the tarsal arch and around bony prominences. When pared with a sharp knife or scalpel the skin surface markings are retained in contrast to the other lesions mentioned.

ii. The cause of these hyperkeratotic lesions is continual minor trauma from ill fitting shoes.

iii. The 'hard skin' needs to be carefully pared off at regular intervals, preferably by a podiatrist. The area needs protection from further trauma and special podiatrists', ring plasters help in this. It is also important to advise that shoes should be comfortable and not rub anywhere on the foot.

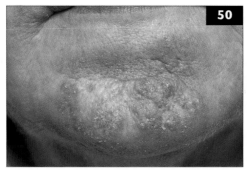

50 A 43-year-old female presents with skin lesions that have appeared in the past 2 months. She has two kinds of lesion: reddened irregular slightly scaling patches (50) on her chin, nose, and forehead, and well-defined firm nodules affecting the cheeks with no changes in the overlying skin.
i. What is the most likely diagnosis and what is the differential diagnosis?
ii. Briefly describe the histopathology of the most likely diagnosis.
iii. Discuss the treatment.

51 A 19-year-old female has had multiple itchy patches on her wrists (51), fingers, ears, and on her trunk in the past 6 months.
i. What is the most likely diagnosis?
ii. How can the diagnosis be confirmed?
iii. What type of immunogical reaction is involved?
iv. Briefly describe the sequence of events.

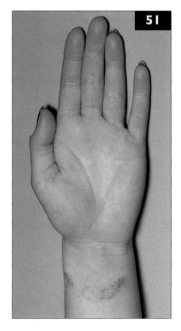

50 i. This patient has both chronic discoid lupus erythematosus (CDLE) and lupus erythematosus profundus lesions. The latter are also known as lupus panniculitis. Lupus panniculitis is quite uncommon and often accompanied by lesions of discoid lupus erythematosus. Other diagnoses that should be considered include sarcoidosis and lymphoma.

ii. Histogically, the picture is to some extent dependent on the type of lesion sampled. There is a striking perivascular accumulation of lymphocytes in the dermis with emphasis on change in the deep dermis and subcutis in the lesions of lupus panniculitis. Areas of necrobiosis are also evident in the deep dermis in lupus panniculitis. Vacuolar change in the basal epidermal layer is present in all cases, but is more evident in the discoid lesions.

iii. Treatment requires experience and patience. The use of topical corticosteroids, especially the very potent agents, is often effective. Chloroquine and hydroxy-chloroquine by mouth are dependable effective suppressive agents. Their use is limited by the toxic side-effect of a macular retinopathy. This is less of a problem with the hydroxychloroquine analogue, but monitoring by ophthalmological experts at regular intervals is still required. Treatment with oral retinoids has been employed for patients with extensive disease. They are quite effective in suppressing the lesions, but are not popular because of the accompanying side-effects. Oral gold compounds and biological agents have also been used.

51 i. The most likely diagnosis is nickel dermatitis. All the sites involved are in contact with a nickel-containing metal article.

ii. The diagnosis is confirmed by a meticulous history and patch testing. A 'standardized test battery' of patches containing the allergens most often found to be the cause of allergic contact dermatitis are applied to the subject's back and kept in place for 48 h. If an area of dermatitis develops at the site of application at 48 h or 72 h (or even 96 h) then the individual is sensitive to the material in that patch.

iii. The reaction, known as allergic contact hypersensitivity, is an example of delayed hypersensitivity or a type IV cellular immune response.

iv. During the initial contact with the skin (induction) the allergen permeates the epidermis and is picked up by the Langerhans cells, which then migrate to the dermis and meet T lymphocytes. These latter then travel to the regional lymph nodes where processing occurs and clones of memory lymphocytes are formed. When the skin subsequently contacts the allergen (elicitation) the lymphocytes migrate to the site of contact on the skin and liberate cytokines, causing an eczematous response locally.

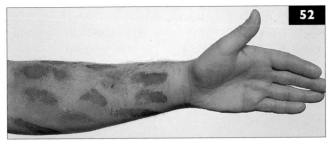

52 The sores on the arms, breasts, and face of this 28-year-old female have been present for the previous 3 years (52). On examination the lesions are oddly shaped erosions. They do not itch a great deal, but do 'weep' at times and the condition is quite 'inconvenient'. The patient worked for 2 years in a publisher's office when she left college, but has not worked since. No treatment has helped. A biopsy does not reveal any specific changes.
i. What is the most likely diagnosis?
ii. How should the condition be managed?

53 A male presents who has had generalized scaling of the skin since he was a baby (53). His sisters are normal.
i. What is the diagnosis?
ii. What disabilities might trouble the patient?
iii. What is the aetiopathogenesis of the condition?

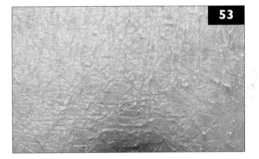

54 A 14-year-old female complains that every year, starting in early spring and remaining troublesome until mid autumn, she has an itchy rash on the face, hands, and arms that seems to be provoked by sun exposure.
i. What investigations should be performed and what findings are to be expected with the most likely diagnosis?
ii. What is the most likely diagnosis and what other diagnoses should be considered?
iii. What management should be recommended?

52 i. The most likely diagnosis is dermatitis artefacta. This condition is considered to be self-induced and presents in a wide variety of guises. In this particular patient it is likely that the erosions were produced by the gouging action of her finger nails. Self-mutilation is always denied by such patients. They often appear curiously indifferent to their condition.

ii. Management is really difficult. Psychiatrists are often reluctant to take on these patients because of their resistance to all forms of treatment. Symptomatic treatment for the lesions should be offered and it is important to provide strong general support.

53 i. The diagnosis is sex-linked ichthyosis. This disorder is transmitted by the female, but manifests only in the male. In many ways it is similar to ordinary autosomal dominant ichthyosis, but tends to be more severe. Histologically, it differs because there is a slight thickening of the epidermal granular cell layer in the sex-linked condition in contrast to an absent granular layer in the autosomal dominant variety.

ii. The appearance is unattractive and because of this there may be social and emotional rejection and isolation. In addition, the inelasticity of the abnormal stratum corneum impedes mobility and fine movements.

iii. The basic metabolic abnormality appears to be a deficiency in the steroid sulphatase enzyme. This alters the ratio of cholesterol sulphate to free cholesterol in the stratum corneum, which in some way causes scaling. This same deficiency prevents the splitting of oestrone sulphate to free oestrone during the last trimester of pregnancy so that the uterus is not 'primed' for the action of oxytocin and parturition is delayed.

54 i. The most likely diagnosis is actinic prurigo. The condition must be distinguished from atopic dermatitis by the absence of sun sensitivity and the presence of high circulating immunoglobulin E (IgE) levels in atopy. It must also be distinguished from erythropoietic protoporphyria and polymorphic light eruption.

ii. There is no single test that will point to the diagnosis. Porphyrin tests and autoantibody tests will be negative. Testing to different wavelengths of light and ultraviolet radiation (UVR) will not reveal a specific hypersensitivity.

iii. Protection from solar irradiation will help, but is not the complete answer – sunscreens certainly do not protect as much as hoped. Steroids may be required and carefully monitored; thalidomide is sometimes helpful.

55 A 27-year-old female presents with a generalized erythematous rash (55) that started just 2 days previously as a few isolated pink patches. In places the skin is blistered and peeling. She feels extremely ill and has to be admitted to a burns unit in a general hospital.
i. What is the most likely diagnosis?
ii. Comment on the possible aetiology.
iii. Discuss the management.

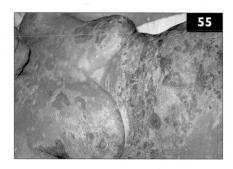

56 i. What is the most likely diagnosis of the lesion in 56?
ii. Are there any disease associations?
iii. What is the recommended management?

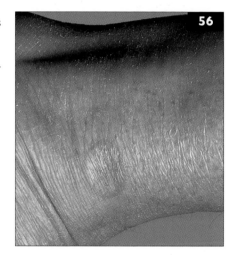

57 A 6-month-old male has had a rash for the past 4 weeks and it is getting worse (57).
i. What is the diagnosis?
ii. What are the main diagnostic features?
iii. What management is recommended?

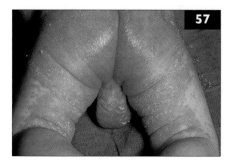

55 i. The most likely diagnosis is toxic epidermal necrolysis. The confluence of the skin lesions and the peeling of sheets of skin distinguishes the disorder from erythema multiforme.

ii. Toxic epidermal necrolysis is of two varieties – the infantile type, which is due to infection with particular toxin-producing serotypes of *Staphyloccus aureus*, and an adult variety due to the administration of drugs such as sulphonamides, some psychotropic agents, and nonsteroidal anti-inflammatory agents. Rarely, no precipitating cause can be found.

iii. There is a high mortality rate of 30–50% and these patients must be treated urgently in a burns unit. Fluid replacement and antibiotics by the intravenous route are necessary interventions, but fastidious nursing care is also of enormous importance. It has been shown that where the disorder is caused by carbamazepine, stopping administration improves the outlook and decreases the severity.

56 i. The most likely diagnosis for the pink annular plaque is granuloma annulare (GA).

ii. The ordinary form of GA is not significantly associated with any particular disorder. The diffuse generalized form, which consists of widespread, flat, multiple lesions, is positively associated with diabetes.

iii. When there are a few localized pink plaques no special treatment is required, as they usually remit spontaneously without sequelae within a few months. More stubborn lesions can be treated with topical or intralesional corticosteroids.

57 i. Primary irritant napkin (diaper) dermatitis is the commonest type of dermatitis in the napkin area. It should be distinguished from infantile seborrhoeic dermatitis, which markedly affects the flexural areas, and from napkin psoriasis, which looks psoriasiform and often affects other areas as well.

ii. The sparing of the flexures, areas of erosion, and a strong smell of ammonia are all typical. This reflects the aetiopathogenesis in which it is thought that urease-secreting bacteria, understandably present in the nappy area, liberate ammonia from the urea of urine, which then causes skin irritation.

iii. The child needs to have its nappy changed more frequently and an emollient should be used. If these measures are not sufficient, 1% hydrocortisone ointment or other weak corticosteroid could be applied twice daily.

58 This 73-year-old male has never had any 'skin trouble', but in recent weeks has begun to complain of an itchy rash on the outer aspects of the upper arms and on the thighs. It is noticed that he has a crepe bandage round his left lower leg. When the elasticated bandage is removed an area of pigmentation redness and scaling is revealed (58).
i. What is the diagnosis?
ii. What investigations should be performed?
iii. What substances are often the cause?

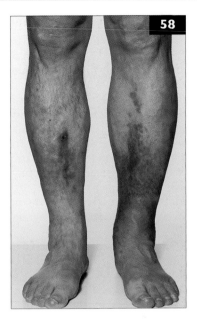

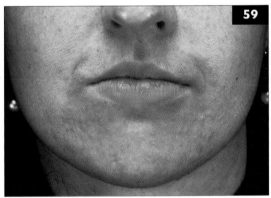

59 Examine the photograph in 59.
i. What is the diagnosis and what is the differential diagnosis?
ii. Comment on the age and sex of the patient.
iii. Discuss the management of such patients.

58 i. The diagnosis is venous eczema with secondary spread. (This used to be called stasis eczema, but the term stasis is inappropriate as, if anything, the rate of blood flow is increased.) Secondary spread to the thighs and upper arms is quite common and is often due to allergic contact dermatitis to one of the medications that have been used.

ii. The only investigation of any help is patch testing. In this, a standard battery of delayed hypersensitivity antigens are placed in occlusive contact with the skin for a 48-h period. The battery of allergens is a set of substances found to be the most frequent causes of allergic contact dermatitis. The sites of application are read shortly after removal of the patches and again at 72 h and if possible 96 h; patches that are persistently and definitely red indicate a positive test reaction to the substance applied to the site.

iii. Patients with venous dermatitis are often found to be sensitive to rubber additives, lanolin, neomycin, fragrances, and microbiocide preservatives.

59 i. The diagnosis is perioral dermatitis. The lesions are typically micropapules or papulopustules. There is a characteristic distribution of lesions around the mouth, leaving a thin uninvolved zone next to the vermillion of the lips. Lesions are also found occasionally around the eyes. There is no background of erythema or telangiectasia and there is no involvement of the cheeks, so rosacea is unlikely. There are no comedones, cysts, or scars and the condition is confined to the lower face, so acne can be excluded.

ii. Perioral dermatitis is predominantly a disease of young females (mostly aged 15–25 years).

iii. Patients with perioral dermatitis should **not** be treated with topical corticosteroids; these agents may temporarily suppress the condition, but it recurs with increased severity within 2 or 3 days of stopping. In fact, no topical agents should be used as they do not help and may aggravate the disease. Patients respond within 3–4 weeks of starting treatment with an oral tetracycline such as doxycycline 50 mg twice daily. Treatment should be continued for 8 weeks and then stopped. Recurrences are rare.

60 A female presents because she thinks that her skin has changed colour. On examination her skin has a golden hue.
i. What is the most likely diagnosis?
ii. What investigations need to be done?
iii. What is the cause of the most likely diagnosis and how is it best managed?

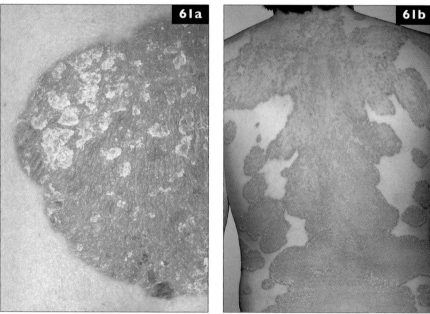

61 A male presents with a scaling rash (61a, b), which is spreading like wildfire! He has had it like this once before, but mostly the problem is kept under control and he generally only suffers from two or three large patches.
i. What is this rash due to?
ii. What problems can it cause?
iii. What management should be recommended?

62 Name and briefly describe risks and discomforts for swimmers from invertebrates.

60 i. The most likely cause of a golden or orange–yellow discolouration of the skin but no systemic associations is the condition of carotenaemia. It is quite different from jaundice or the brownish discolouration due to haemachromatosis.
ii. Blood levels of beta carotene need to be performed.
iii. The condition is due to eating large quantities of beta carotene-containing foods – carrots in particular. The best management is to persuade the patient to give up the habit of eating large numbers of carrots!

61 i. The rash is due to psoriasis. Other conditions that cause a generalized and rapidly spreading rash include drug eruptions, severe generalized eczema, skin lymphoma, and pityriasis rubra pilaris.
ii. The generalized erythema can result in hypothermia from the loss of heat and the increased blood supply to the skin results in a high cardiac output state and may even result in high output failure. The disturbance of the skin barrier causes increased transepidermal water loss and dehydration. Such patients are also socially and occupationally profoundly disabled.
iii. Patients affected to this extent need to be at rest and kept warm, even though because of their warm skin they may appear to have a fever; it is also important to ensure that they do not become dehydrated. Initially, the only topical treatments required are emollients. Subsequently patients may need treatment with methotrexate, ciclosporin, photochemotherapy with ultraviolet A (PUVA), retinoids, or biological agents such as etanercept or infliximab.

62 i. Jellyfish stings are intensely painful areas where skin contact has occurred with the trailing tentacles of jellyfish. The condition is due to discharge of tiny nematocysts. The pain and discomfort last up to 2 h.
ii. Cercarial dermatitis (swimmer's itch) is due to cercarial larvae from schistosoma species that do not normally parasitize humans. They cause an unpleaseant itch and are a problem of some freshwater lakes.
iii. Sea urchin granuloma is skin injury sustained from sea urchin spines in tropical seas. Retained spines cause persistent swollen red areas due to granulomatous inflammation.
iv. Cutaneous larva migrans is caused by invasion of skin by the larvae of hookworms that do not usually parasitize humans. It is sustained commonly on Caribbean beaches. The larvae produce meandering itchy red tracks in the skin of the buttocks and back in particular.

63 A 15-year-old female presents with a widespread rash. The spots have been there for the last 3 weeks and are still spreading; the larger ones now have scales on the surface (63). The problem started after the patient had a sore throat about 5 or 6 weeks previously. She had one previous similar attack at the age of 12 years, which eventually cleared spontaneously.
i. What is the differential diagnosis?
ii. Briefly discuss the aetiopathogenesis of the most likely diagnosis.
iii. Briefly discuss the management.

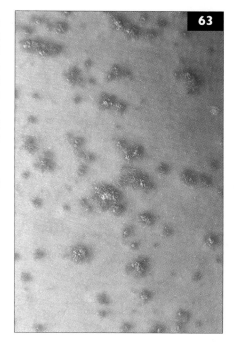

64 This 64-year-old patient's rash (64) was first treated as ringworm even though it had been present unchanging for several months.
i. What is the differential diagnosis?
ii. What investigations would help establish the diagnosis?
iii. What is your treatment plan for this patient?

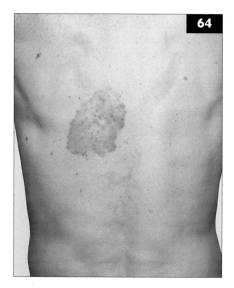

63 i. The list of possible diagnoses includes guttate psoriasis, pityriasis rosea, secondary syphilis, viral exanthem, drug eruption, and early stages of human immunodeficiency virus (HIV) disease. The spots are well-defined, slightly raised, and scaling – these characteristics and the history make guttate psoriasis the most likely diagnosis.

ii. The molecular basis for psoriasis is still uncertain, but guttate psoriasis is provoked by beta-haemolytic streptococcal throat infections. It is thought that an erythemogenic toxin of the bacteria sets off the psoriatic process.

iii. Throat swabs should be taken to determine whether the beta-haemolytic *Streptococcus* is still present. If it is, a full course of penicillin should be given. The rash itself does not often require heroic treatment as the condition usually spontaneously remits after some weeks or months. Emollients, weak salicylic acid and tar preparations, and weak corticosteroid preparations may be used. Uncommonly, the rash is stubborn and requires phototherapy.

64 i. The condition was unlikely to be due to ringworm as it was persistent, evolved too slowly, was figurate and not annular, and did not respond to antifungal agents. The patch was 'solitary' and on close examination had a fine hair-like raised margin. These characteristics suggest that the lesion is a superficial basal cell carcinoma. Other disorders giving rise to red scaling patches include psoriasis, eczema, Bowen's disease (intraepidermal epithelioma), and skin lymphoma. Determining the right diagnosis can sometimes be quite difficult.

ii. Examination of surface scales microscopically for fungal mycelium after treating the sample with 20% potassium hydroxide is an important way of excluding ringworm. Biopsy and subsequent histological examination will reveal the characteristic changes of basal cell carcinoma and distinguish the lesion from Bowen's disease, psoriasis, and eczema.

iii. The treatment depends on the site and the size of the lesion, as well as the preference of the patient. Surgical excision is the most certain technique, but by no means always possible. Curettage is often used and is the most suitable treatment in many patients. Increasing use is being made of 5% imiquimod cream. This immunomodulating agent successfully ablates 75% of lesions after 6 weeks of use.

65 A female is extremely embarrassed at the excessive sweating of her palms, axillae, and forehead.
i. What is this condition called and what are its main features?
ii. What disabilities can it cause?
iii. Outline the main approaches to treatment.

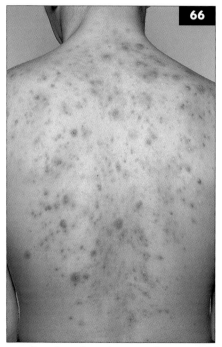

66 A 19-year-old unemployed male, who spends most of his time at the gym, complains of a recent worsening of his acne with many large painful lesions on his face and upper back (66).
i. What explanations are possible for the sudden worsening of his acne?
ii. Describe the pathology of an acne cyst.
iii. What management should be recommended for his acne?

65 i. The condition is known as hyperhidrosis. It is mainly a problem for individuals in the second and third decades of life. The areas most often affected by the excessive sweating are the palms, soles, axillae, and forehead, but other sites are also involved in some patients. The affected areas sweat with emotional stimuli and spontaneously, but not with heat.

ii. Sweating palms make hand shaking and any other type of skin contact embarrassing. It is also difficult to write on paper because of the degree of wetness of the palms. The underarm sweating produces unsightly damp patches and, if severe enough, causes clothes to rot. Excess sweating of the feet causes embarrassing malodour and may cause shoes to rot.

iii. Mildly affected individuals may respond to aluminium hexachlorhydrate in high concentrations in stick form or lotion. Anticholinergic drugs sometimes help. Iontophoresis in solutions of povidone methanesulphonate, or even plain water, seems to assist some patients, but is associated with several adverse side-effects. Sympathectomy has been used for severely affected patients. In recent years subcutaneous injections of botulinum toxin at affected sites have been used to control sweating for a period of some months.

66 i. One possible explanation for the worsening of his acne is that the patient has been taking anabolic steroids. These are taken not infrequently by 'body builders' and are well known to aggravate acne. Another possibility is that the sudden worsening is due to the condition of acne fulminans. In this unpleasant and little understood complication of acne, existing lesions become larger and more inflamed and more lesions develop. In addition, there is malaise and leucoytosis and, in some patients, arthropathy and splenomegaly.

ii. An acne cyst is not really a cyst at all, but a 'cold abscess' in which a central cavity is filled with tissue debris and dead inflammatory cells.

iii. Patients with severe cystic acne should be treated with the standard course of isotretinoin (0.5–1.0 mg/kg daily PO) over a 4-month period. If they are unwell and have many very inflamed lesions then many advocate a course of prednisolone at the same time. Antibiotics and dapsone are also sometimes used.

67 This red plaque-like condition (67) has a 'velvety' surface. It has been present for the past 6 months and is slowly spreading.
i. What is the likely diagnosis?
ii. Briefly describe the possible disorders that may cause this appearance.
iii. Briefly outline the plan for management of this patient.

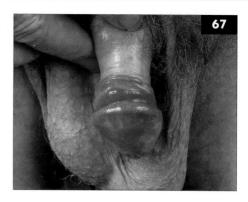

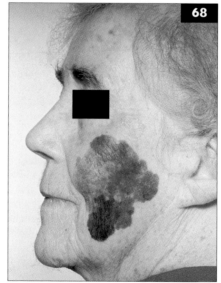

68 A female presents with a brown–black patch which has become increasingly noticeable in the past 5 years. It is covering an increasing area on her left cheek and is becoming darker in some places (68).
i. What is the diagnosis?
ii. What treatments are available for this disease?
iii. What type of person is usually affected?

67 i. The most likely diagnosis is the precancerous condition of erythroplasia of Queyrat. The main differential diagnosis is the inflammatory dermatosis known as Zoon's balanitis. This can mimic the precancerous condition clinically, but is easily distinguishable histologically by the presence of large numbers of plasma cells and haemosiderin pigment and the absence of cellular atypia. Patches of eczema and psoriasis can resemble erythroplasia, but there usually are patches elsewhere as well.

ii. Erythroplasia of Queyrat is a form of intraepidermal epithelioma (a type of Bowen's disease). In many instances one of the antigenic strains of the human papillomavirus (HPV) can be recovered from affected tissue (HPV16 and HPV18 being examples). The condition has a characteristic appearance as a well-defined red plaque with a shiny glazed surface. Zoon's balanitis may look quite similar to erythroplasia, although it may have a slightly brownish tinge. It is thought to be a response to infection, but its aetiopathogensis is uncertain.

iii. The first step in management is to make a definitive diagnosis and a biopsy is often required for this purpose. Histologically, erythroplasia of Queyrat resembles Bowen's disease with marked cellular atypia and epidermal thickening. Oncogenic human papillomaviruses can be identified in, and recovered from, the large majority of lesions of erythroplasia of Queyrat. It is thought to be similar to the condition of Bowenoid papulosis and there is a strong risk of onward progression to squamous cell carcinoma (30% in some estimates). Histologically, Zoon's balanitis shows a subepidermal inflammatory infiltrate composed largely of plasma cells. Erythroplasia is treated surgically if possible or with topical chemotherapy (5-fluorouracil or imiquimod); Zoon's balanitis is treated by circumcision, hygiene measures, and topical antimicrobials or antimicrobial–corticosteroid combinations.

68 i. The diagnosis is most likely to be lentigo maligna, also known as Hutchinson's freckle, precancerous melanosis of Dubreuil, and melanoma *in situ*. The main differential diagnosis is seborrhoeic wart – which can look worryingly like lentigo maligna – the slight surface roughness or wartiness and fawn or light brown pigmentation being important distinguishing features of a seborrhoeic wart.

ii. Excision is recommended, but because of its site and size this may not be possible. Radiotherapy is strongly advocated by some. Other less effective treatments include 20% azelaic acid cream topically twice daily over several weeks or months and 3% imiquimod cream three times a week over 3 or 4 weeks.

iii. The affected individual is usually elderly, fair complexioned, and often quite sun damaged.

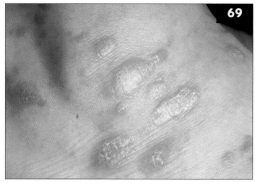

69 i. What are the lesions in 69?
ii. Where else might signs of this disorder be found?
iii. Is this disease known to have particular associations with other disorders?

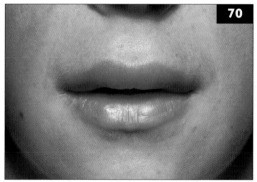

70 A male has had three attacks in which his lips and tongue became swollen (70), each attack lasting about 8 h.
i. What is this disorder? Are there any serious consequences of this condition?
ii. What are the common causes of this disorder?
iii. Briefly outline the management.

71 i. What are the causes of acquired immunosuppression?
ii. What specific skin problems may be encountered by someone who has had a renal transplant?
iii. Briefly describe the dermatological management of a patient who has had a renal transplant.

69 i. The disorder is lichen planus. The flat-topped, often polygonal-shaped, mauve papules are typical of this disease. Lesions can occur anywhere, but are particularly common on the front of the wrist and over the back. They are often extremely pruritic.

ii. The buccal mucosa is often affected with a whitish network or, less frequently, white spots. Other mucosae (e.g. vaginal) are occasionally affected. If the nails are affected, destruction of the nail plate and scarring may occur, but more commonly vertical striations develop alone. If the scalp is affected, areas of hair loss with scarring are seen.

iii. Lichen planus appears to be autoimmune in origin and a variety of other autoimmune disorders have been described as being associated, including lupus erythematosus, bullous pemphigoid, rheumatoid arthritis, and biliary cirrhosis.

70 i. Sudden swelling of the lips, tongue, and other soft tissues of the head and neck region is characteristic of angioedema. It lasts a few hours before subsiding. It is occasionally accompanied by urticarial weals over the skin of the trunk and limbs. If the soft tissues of the fauces are affected, there may be difficulty in breathing, even leading to suffocation and death.

ii. The condition is caused by immediate hypersensitivity to various allergens including peanuts, penicillin, and wasp and bee stings. It is also a feature of a congenital disorder in which there is a deficiency of a constituent of the complement cascade known as the C1 esterase inhibitor.

iii. The most important issues in the management are the identification of the precipitating allergen by a detailed history, intracutaneous tests (prick tests) using a battery of common allergens, and blood tests to assay the complement components. Avoidance of exposure to the allergen is also important. Regular administration of prophylactic antihistamines may help. Carrying around loaded syringes containing 1 in 1000 epinephrine (adrenaline) to be self-administered by intramuscular injection may be life saving.

71 i. Immunosuppression may be drug induced or due to disease. Drugs causing immunosuppression include glucocorticoids (e.g. prednisolone), ciclosporin, methotrexate, and azathroprine and they are usually admistered for their immunosuppressive effects.

ii. Transplant patients are prone to solar keratoses, Bowen's disease, squamous cell carcinoma, malignant melanoma, and Kaposi's sarcoma. They are also vulnerable to viral warts, molluscum contagiosum, and fungal infections.

iii. Such patients must be urged to protect themselves from the sun and to attend follow-up clinics to check on early lesions.

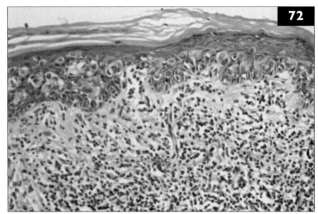

72 i. What are the possible origins of the clear cells within the epidermis in 72?
ii. The biopsy comes from a red scaling patch in the groin area of a 63-year-old male. What is the most likely diagnosis?
iii. Does this diagnosis have any important clinical associations?
iv. What management is recommended?

73 A male presents with a problem with his hands that started about 8 weeks after his company had introduced a new lubricant for the machines on which he works. He has been a machine minder for 12 years and has not had a problem previously. The rash affects both hands, with extension onto the left wrist (73). There is no rash elsewhere on his skin. The rash fluctuates in intensity with episodes of vesiculation, weeping, and cracking, but seems to clear at weekends.
i. What is the likely cause of this skin disorder?
ii. What disabilities would the patient have?
iii. Discuss the management for this patient.

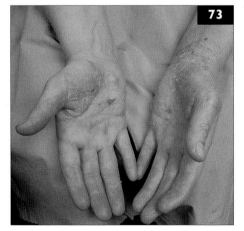

72 i. The large clear cells could be Paget cells (either from mammary Paget's disease or extramammary Paget's disease [EMPD]), abnormal keratinocytes in Bowen's disease cells, abnormal melanocytes in superficial spreading melanoma, or abnormal T lymphocytes in mycosis fungoides.

ii. Given the histological appearance, the red scaling patch in the groin is due either to EMPD or Bowen's disease. As the lesion is in the perigenital area of a man and is not psoriasisform clinically or histologically, it is most likely to be due to EMPD.

iii. EMPD is associated with neoplastic disease of the apocrine glands in the underlying skin or, occasionally, with neoplastic lesions in organs further afield such as the rectum, the bladder, or the prostate.

iv. The management is to look for any underlying neoplasm, remove it if one is found, and to remove the affected area of the skin surgically.

73 i. The rash is most likely to be an occupationally-induced hand eczema (dermatitis). The weeping is more like eczema than psoriasis and the absence of skin involvement elsewhere is also supportive of the diagnosis of eczema. The major site of involvement (the hands) is also in favour of the disorder being occupationally determined.

ii. Such a skin disorder would cause major problems. The pain and discomfort prevent use of the hands for everyday domestic and social tasks, and work. In addition, the rash on his hands inhibits friends, colleagues, and relatives as far as close contact is concerned.

iii. The patient needs to be patch tested to ensure that he does not have a contact sensitivity and it is advisable that he be seen in a department that is familiar with this technique. He will need to have the standard 'European patch test battery' of allergens applied as well as any suspected materials (in suitable dilution). He will need to avoid handling irritant materials and working with his hands until several weeks after they are healed. Emollients are important and these, combined with topical corticosteroids (starting with weak or moderate strength preparations), form the mainstay of treatment.

74 This patient's acne had been quite troublesome in his teenage years, but now at the age of 22 it has largely cleared, except for the firm lumpy swellings on his upper back (74). These have been there for the past 18 months and, if anything, seem to have increased in size.

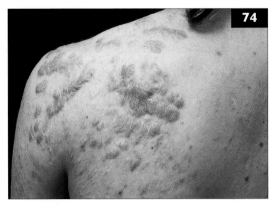

i. What is the diagnosis?
ii. Are any groups especially prone to this condition?
iii. How should the condition be managed?

75 A 27-year-old female complains that at regular intervals of 3 or 4 weeks she develops sore red patches on her skin (75). The patches always occur at the same sites. Sometimes the patches blister. When they fade they leave pigmented areas.
i. What is the diagnosis?
ii. How can the diagnosis be confirmed?
iii. Briefly describe the management.

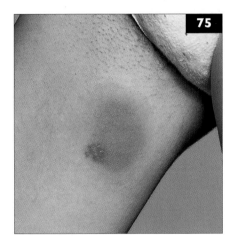

76 A male presents with brownish, warty streaks that seem to be becoming more prominent every year. He is concerned about their appearance.
i. What is the diagnosis?
ii. What might a biopsy reveal?
iii. Discuss the management of this condition.

74 i. These are keloid scars. Many kinds of trauma can precipitate keloid scars, but severe acne is one of the most frequent causes.

ii. Young people (particularly young women) aged 12–24 years are the most often affected and individuals of African ancestry are affected more frequently than other racial groups.

iii. There are many different treatments for keloid scars. Simple excision and suturing often results in recurrence of the keloid. Intracutaneous injection with a potent steroid (triamcinolone acetonide or methylprednisolone) is sometimes successful, but is difficult to control and can result in skin atrophy. A combination of excision and steroid injection has been used with inconsistent results. Injections of collagenase and gamma interferon have been used with variable results. Radiotherapy and the administration of infliximab have also been used with variable results.

75 i. The patient is suffering from a fixed drug eruption. The history of a recurrent rash in which inflamed and sometimes blistered lesions always appear at the same sites then fade and leave a pigmented stain is quite typical. It is sometimes difficult to discover the drug responsible; in this case it was mefenamic acid taken for dysmenorrhoea on a monthly basis.

ii. It is important to be certain about the diagnosis and it is often considered prudent, after consultation with the patient, to administer the suspected drug in a challenge test. A biopsy of the rash will reveal changes similar to those seen in erythema multiforme, with perivascular mononuclear cell infiltrate also involving the epidermis.

iii. Having established the diagnosis the drug should be prohibited. Care must also be taken with drugs of a similar chemical structure. During an acute attack the lesions may be treated with topical corticosteroids.

76 i. Epidermal naevus.

ii. Biopsy often shows regular epidermal thickening with a 'church spire' architecture. In a small proportion of cases the epidermis shows the same kind of degenerative change as in the rare dominantly inherited type of ichthyosis known as epidermolytic hyperkeratosis.

iii. If the lesion is small enough, surgical excision is the best form of management. Alternatively, keratolytics (salicylic acid- or tretinoin-containing topical agents) can help.

77 i. What is the condition illustrated in 77?
ii. What is known of its aetiopathogenesis?
iii. Describe the pathology of the condition.

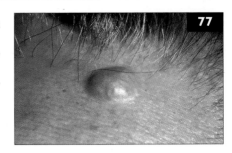

78 A 27-year-old male complains of a red rash on the palms, which started 10 months previously and is gradually worsening (78). It does not blister and is not itchy but is cracked and painful. It is persistent and none of the treatments he has used have helped.
i. What is the most likely diagnosis and what is the differential diagnosis?
ii. What accompanying signs would assist in confirming the diagnosis?
iii. Describe a suitable treatment regimen and an alternative to this.

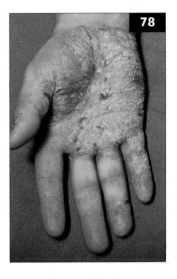

79 i. What is this condition (79)?
ii. What are the clinical features of this disorder?
iii. What is the molecular basis of the disease?

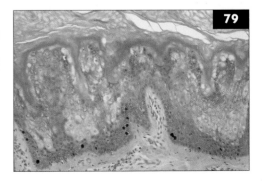

77 i. The condition is cylindroma (turban tumour). It is characterized by the development of solitary or, more often, multiple, rounded, pink or flesh-coloured benign tumours on the scalp.
ii. The lesions are thought to be derived from sweat gland epithelium and to be inherited as an autosomal dominant characteristic.
iii. The tumours consist of lobules containing small basophilic cells at the periphery with paler cells centrally. Surrounding the lobules is an eosinophilic hyaline material.

78 i. The most likely diagnosis is psoriasis. This can be very difficult to distinguish from chronic eczema of the hands, although hand eczema tends to be more itchy and to blister. Chronic ringworm usually affects one palm and is more scaly and less inflamed than psoriasis.
ii. The presence of psoriasis elsewhere (e.g. knees, elbows, and scalp), would be quite supportive of a diagnosis of psoriasis of the palms, as would nail pitting or other sign of nail involvement.
iii. Potent topical corticosteroids together with either vitamin D analogues (such as calcipotriol) or topical retinoids (e.g. tazarotene) are often used as topical agents. An alternative treatment would be the use of photochemotherapy with long-wave ultraviolet radiation (UVA) and an oral or topical psoralen. Severely affected individuals may require oral treatments such as acitretin, methotrexate, or ciclosporin. In the most intractable cases biologicals, such as etanercept or infliximab, should be considered.

79 i. This appearance of a vesicular reticular degenerate change in the upper epidermis is pathognomonic of epidermolytic hyperkeratosis, also known as bullous ichthyosiform erythroderma.
ii. There are three main types – the most common is the generalized type. This and a type confined to the palms and soles are inherited as autosomal dominant characteristics. A third and rare type occurs sporadically in localized naevoid patches. The condition is characterized by hyperkeratosis, erythema, and a tendency to blister.
iii. The molecular basis is a mutation in certain keratin genes (keratin 5 and keratin 9) interfering with the formation of tonofibrils.

80 An obese 54-year-old female presents with a rash beneath both her breasts. She also has a rash affecting her scalp, buttocks, and knees, which, like the rash beneath her breasts, is red, slightly raised and scaling, and has a well-defined margin. There is no history of skin disorder in the family.
i. What is the diagnosis?
ii. What else could the condition be?
iii. Describe an appropriate treatment regimen and one other treatment if the first does not work.

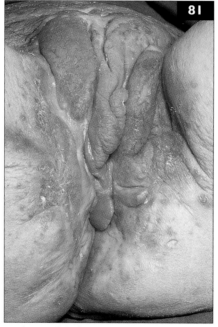

81 A patient presents with painful abscesses and draining sinuses that have recurred in the axillae and groins on an irregular basis over the previous 10 years (81) and do not respond to antibiotics.
i. What is the diagnosis?
ii. What is the current view as to the pathogenesis of this condition?
iii. Briefly describe the management.

71

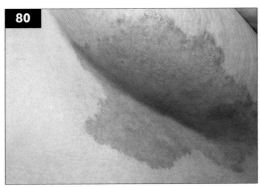

80 i. The diagnosis is flexural psoriasis. The well-defined edge, the symmetry, and the presence of a similar rash on her knees and scalp much favour this diagnosis (80).
ii. Other possibilities include intertrigo, leading to infectious eczematoid dermatitis, and ringworm.
iii. The patient should avoid exertion and remain resting until the condition is improved. She should not wear tight underwear. Gentle bathing with normal saline twice daily with application of a moderately potent corticosteroid cream after patting dry is indicated. If this treatment does not succeed in suppressing the condition, systemic therapy such as methotrexate, ciclosporin, or biological agents may need to be considered.

81 i. The diagnosis is hidradenitis suppurativa. The condition may be very disabling because of the pain and constantly draining sinuses.
ii. It used to be thought that the disorder was due to inflammation affecting the apocrine glands. This is now disputed and it is believed that the whole pilosebaceous unit is involved. The condition is thought of as being similar to acne (an acne equivalent). The type of initiating event is uncertain.
iii. Unfortunately, drug treatments are not often successful – tetracyclines (as for acne), isotretinoin (as for acne), and dapsone have all been used. In recent years some success has been reported for infliximab. The most successful treatment is the total extirpation of all hair and sweat units and surrounding soft tissues from the affected areas in the axillae and groins. The surgery leaves unpleasant scarring, but is appreciated by the patients because of the relief from the draining sinuses.

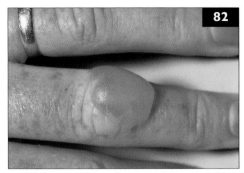

82 A female presents with blistering confined to the backs of her hands (82) and her forehead. She is taking captopril and furosemide to control her blood pressure.
i. Suggest the cause of her blistering rash.
ii. Discuss the histological appearances of the condition.
iii. What is the prognosis and what management should be recommended?

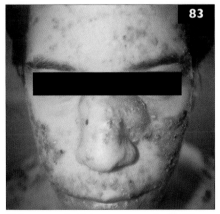

83 i. What is the condition seen in this young male (83)?
ii. He says that it developed quite suddenly. What are the possible explanations for this?
iii. What management should be recommended?

82 i. The cause of the blistering rash is the furosemide diuretic the patient was taking to control her blood pressure. This drug-induced disorder is known as pseudoporphyria because of its apparent similarity to porphyria cutanea tarda. Interestingly, captopril can also produce a blistering rash, but this is more often pemphigus like.

ii. Blistering that occurs in the pattern of porphyria cutanea tarda (pseudo-porphyria) is subepidermal. Blistering due to captopril may cause a pemphigus-like disease and, histologically, acantholysis and suprabasilar cresting are seen.

iii. The blisters will cease to develop when the causative drug is changed. The individual blistered areas only require simple topical treatment with nonadherent dressings.

83 i. The condition is severe nodulocystic acne. Note that there are many large inflammatory lesions – large papules, nodules, and cysts.

ii. Sudden worsening of acne together with the appearances of cysts is seen as an unexplained occurrence and may be accompanied by malaise, high leucocytosis, and painful joints in the condition known as acne fulminans. There may also be splenomegaly and punched out rarefactions at the end of long bones. Sudden worsening of acne occurs in weight lifters and body builders illegally taking anabolic steroids (such as stanozolol). It is seen in those poisoned by dioxin and similar compounds after industrial accidents. Sudden worsening of acne is also seen in soldiers in the wet tropics; sudden flares of acne was a not uncommon cause of evacuation of young soldiers from Vietnam.

iii. Management may be complex and is dependent on the cause. Antibiotics in full dosage (usually doxycycline or erythromycin) are given. A short course of prednisolone (40–60 mg daily) is often added. A course of isotretinoin is also started once the early severe inflammatory stage has passed.

84 The upper face of a child who complains bitterly that his eyes itch is shown (84).
i. What is this condition?
ii. What other sites on the body are often affected by this disease?
iii. Are there any ophthalmological complications in this disorder?
iv. What treatments might be appropriate for a patient with severe chronic generalized atopic dermatitis?

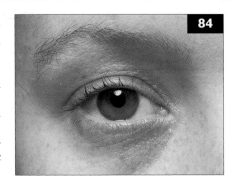

85 It is never easy to determine the cause of focal scalp hair loss.
i. What is the differential diagnosis of the hair loss in the patient in 85?
ii. What investigations would assist in reaching the correct diagnosis?
iii. Discuss the management of the most likely diagnosis.

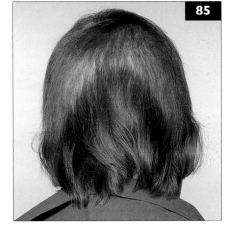

86 A 55-year-old male presents with fatigue and recent pain and discolouration of his right lower leg; there are a few scattered ecchymoses and his gums are swollen and inflamed. He is a somewhat odd and isolated character and has not made much progress professionally or socially.
i. What is the most likely diagnosis?
ii. What other physical signs may accompany the disorder?
iii. How may the diagnosis be confirmed?
iv. How should the condition be treated?

84 i. This condition is classical atopic dermatitis. The line or crease beneath the eyes is known as a Denny–Morgan fold. The paucity of eyebrows and eyelashes results from continual rubbing, as does the dark shadowing of the skin around the eyes. Surrounding skin tends to be pale and slightly scaly.
ii. The antecubital fossae, the popliteal fossae, the wrists, and the sides of the neck are the other sites most often affected.
iii. Keratomalacia leading to keratoconus and even corneal perforation are one group of associated ophthalmic problems. Cataracts are also a rare complication, but it is uncertain whether the disease itself or its treatment with topical corticosteroids is the cause of these cataracts.
iv. Systemic drugs, such as azathioprine, ciclosporin, tacrolimus, or steroids, may be necessary. Phototherapy is also used on occasion.

85 i. The presence of broken hairs and the irregular shape of the hairless area suggest a diagnosis of trichitillomania. If it is established that the affected area is not scarred, the other diagnoses that need serious consideration are aloepecia areata and tinea capitis.
ii. Investigations that may help in reaching the correct diagnosis include examination of hair clippings and skin scrapings for ringworm fungus. Skin biopsy will also give important information.
iii. In this patient's case the most likely diagnosis is that of trichitillomania and unfortunately the management of this self-inflicted disorder is difficult. Psychiatric advice should be sought – but is rarely of much help. Luckily, the tendency to pull out hair does eventually pass in most patients.

86 i. The most likely diagnosis is scurvy. This is seen in isolated individuals who have had an inadequate diet over recent months with little or no fruit and vegetables.
ii. Follicular hyperkeratosis, perifollicular haemorrhages, xeroderma, and arthropathy are amongst the frequent concomitant findings in scurvy.
iii. Measurement of serum ascorbate levels before and after administration of a loading dose of ascorbic acid has been recommended as a confirmatory test, but it is rarely done in practice.
iv. The condition should be treated with vitamin C and care should be directed towards correcting any poor dietary habits.

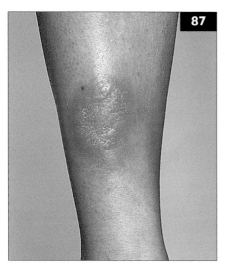

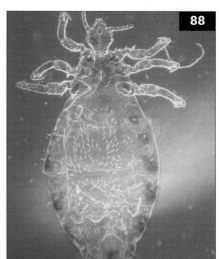

87 i. What is this plaque-like condition (87) that has affected both shins, worse on the right, in the past 6 months? The lesions have gradually enlarged over this period.
ii. Are there other physical features that sometimes develop in this disease?
iii. Briefly outline the pathogenesis of this condition.

88 i. What is this creature (88)?
ii. Where does it live? How is it spread?
iii. What is the treatment of choice?
iv. Are there similar parasites that afflict humans?

89 A 6-month-old baby girl presents with a rash on the face and truncal flexures. It looks like seborrhoeic dermatitis and is accompanied by a slight fever and signs of general unwellness.
i. What is the differential diagnosis and what is the most likely diagnosis?
ii. Briefly describe the pathogenesis and the pathology of the most likely diagnosis.
iii. Briefly describe the management of this patient.

87 i. This disorder, recognized by its plaque-like appearance and peau d'orange appearance on the surface, is pretibial myxoedema (PTM).
ii. PTM is part of a more widespread disorder characterized by exophthalmos, clubbing of the finger nails, and soft tissue thickening of the hands known as thyroid acropachy.
iii. There is a circulating peptide in this disorder, which has the ability to stimulate fibroblast growth *in vitro*. PTM is always associated with thyrotoxicosis.

88 i. The creature in the illustration is a head louse (*Pediculus humanus capitis*).
ii. It lives on the scalp, attached tightly by its claws to the hair shaft. When necessary it scuttles down to the scalp skin for a meal of human blood. It lays eggs (nits) that are stuck to the hair shaft. It is spread by head-to-head or hair-to-hair contact.
iii. The treatment of choice is with phenothrin (0.2% or 0.5%) lotion or emulsion. The preparation is rubbed into the scalp, allowed to dry and then shampooed out after 12 h. Another treatment is with malathion 0.5%, which is rubbed into the scalp and allowed to dry for 12 h before shampooing. The application is repeated after 7 days. Some advise use of a nit comb as well.
iv. *Phthirus pubis* (the crab louse) is a related parasite that causes pubic infestations. It is spread by sexual contact.

89 i. A likely diagnosis is class I histiocytosis (the older name for this is Letterer–Siwe disease). Characteristically, the appearance is of an erythematosquamous, sometimes papular rash on the face and trunk in the flexural sites, looking a little like seborrhoeic dermatitis. It may be associated with some systemic pulmonary, hepatosplenic, and bony involvement in a small proportion of patients, and the disorder can have a fatal outcome. Seborrhoeic dermatitis or a transient exanthem should be considered in the differential diagnosis.
ii. The disorder is essentially the result of a benign proliferation of marrow-derived histocytic cells that invade the epidermis and are destined to become Langerhans cells. Histologically, collections of large mononuclear cells containing Birbeck granules ultrastructurally (typical of Langerhans cells) are found within the epidermis or in the papillary dermis.
iii. The disorder ranges from a mild disturbance to a severe and even fatal illness and the management will depend on the severity in the individual patient. Topical nitrogen mustard and psoralen plus ultraviolet phototherapy have been employed for extensive cutaneous lesions; systemic steroids, methotrexate, and 6-mercapto-purine, as well as other antimitotic agents, have been used when the disorder affects several organ systems.

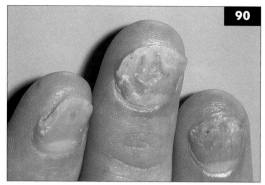

90 i. What is wrong with this person's nails (90)? Should any other disorder be considered?
ii. How might one try to confirm the diagnosis.
iii. Briefly describe the problems that might arise from such a disorder.

91 A 35-year-old female has had attacks of facial flushing over the past few months. She has also had attacks of diarrhoea and wheezing.
i. What is a likely diagnosis?
ii. Briefly describe the pathogenesis of the most likely diagnosis.
iii. Discuss complications of the disorder.
iv. Is there a biochemical test for this disease?

92 A patient presents with multiple skin papules; the papules are pink, excoriated and, in many cases umbilicated or crusted. They seem to have slowly evolved over a 6-month period and are mostly situated over the limbs. A biopsy shows an unusal feature – the presence of damaged collagen bundles, which from their position and orientation appear to be in the process of expulsion to the exterior.
i. What is the likely diagnosis?
ii. What is the name of the group of diseases showing this type of perforating process or transepidermal elimination?
iii. Name at least two other skin disorders in which a similar kind of elimination process is seen.
iv. Are there any conditions that predispose to this disorder?

90 i. The patient is suffering from psoriasis. The nail plates are thickened and yellowish and there is subungual debris. The finger nails also show pitting and patches of pink and green–black discolouration. The main differential diagnosis is tinea unguium and, on the toe nails, the two conditions are really quite hard to differentiate.

ii. Absence of fungal mycelium in nail clippings is important. The presence of psoriasis elsewhere on the skin and/or the presence of psoriasis in a first-degree relative would tend to support the diagnosis.

iii. Psoriasis of the toe nails gives rise to very few problems. However, psoriasis of the finger nails causes major cosmetic problems, which may cause serious issues in patients who need 'good looking' hands, such as waiters and waitresses and shop assistants. Abnormal nails may also interfere with fine finger movement causing problems for those who work with instruments or are musicians.

91 i. A likely diagnosis is the carcinoid syndrome. This is the result of a tumour of neuroendocine cells (Argentaffin cells), which may affect the gastrointestinal tract or the bronchi. It is said that up to 5% of patients who complain of recent onset of flushing may suffer from the carcinoid syndrome.

ii. Carcinoid tumours secrete vasoactive substances, particularly 5-hydroxytryptamine (serotonin), but also substance P, bradykinin, and histamine. The majority of carcinoid tumours are found incidentally at autopsy. Generally, systemic symptoms do not occur until the amount of vasoactive material produced and secreted outweighs the liver's capacity to detoxify it. In most cases systemic symptoms occur when liver metastases develop.

iii. Pellagra, a manifestation of nicotinamide deficiency, may develop due to deviation of tryptophan from nicotinamide synthesis into 5-hydroxytryptamine synthesis. Right-sided heart disease may develop due to fibrosis around the tricuspid valve and elsewhere. True rosacea has been recorded on rare occasions in patients who flush particularly dramatically.

iv. The biochemical test available is the measurement of urinary 5-hydroxyindo-leacetic acid.

92 i. A likely diagnosis is acquired reactive perforating collagenosis.

ii. The group of diseases showing similar changes is the perforating disorders and the process is sometimes known as transepidermal elimination.

iii. Other examples of perforating disorders include elastosis perforans serpiginosa and granuloma annulare.

iv. Diabetes mellitus, renal disease, and hepatic disorders seem to predispose to acquired reactive perforating collagenosis.

93 A photomicrograph of a biopsy from a 48-year-old female with a 2-month history of an itchy maculopapular rash of the trunk is shown (93).
i. What is the diagnosis?
ii. What are the characteristic histological features?
iii. Is there a specific variety of this disorder that occurs in men?
iv. Is there an effective treatment?

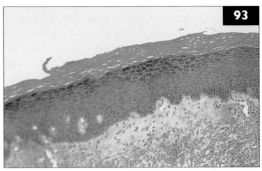

94 A male presents after being teased about his nose (94). It has enlarged irregularly and become discoloured in the past 2–3 years.
i. What is the diagnosis?
ii. What disorder(s) is it associated with?
iii. Briefly describe the histopathological appearance of this condition.
iv. Discuss the treatment.

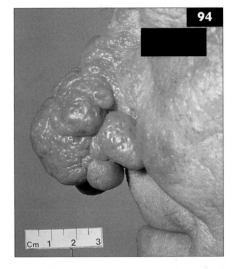

95 A male presents with odd marks on his legs and is feeling unwell. He had been camping some 2 weeks previously and said he had quite a lot of insect bites including what seemed to be tick bites.
i. What is a likely diagnosis?
ii. Briefly describe the cause and the epidemiology of this disorder.
iii. What are some of the other clinical manifestations of this disease.
iv. What tests are available to confirm the diagnosis.

93 i. The diagnosis is lichen sclerosus et atrophicus (white spot disease).
ii. The intensely oedematous band subepidermally, the slight epidermal thickening but basal cell liquefactive degenerative change; the perivascular lymphocytic cuffing.
iii. A scarring disorder in men appears particularly on the glans penis and is known as balanitis xerotica obliterans.
iv. Application of clobetasol propionate ointment has been reported to induce remission.

94 i. The diagnosis is rhinophyma. Rarely, sarcoidosis or some form of neoplastic disease can simulate the condition. The irregular thickening and the dull red–mauve discolouration are typical.
ii. Rhinophyma is mostly observed as a complication of rosacea. It is no longer thought to be the result of alcoholism. Uncommonly, it may occur as a complication of chronic severe acne. It also may occur in isolation unassociated with any other condition.
iii. The histopathology is charcterized by the presence of hypertrophied sebaceous glands, many large ectatic vascular channels, dense mixed inflammatory cell infiltrate, and early fibrosis.
iv. Topical medications and systemic tetracyclines have no effect. Systemic isotretinoin may shrink the nose while the drug is administered because of its effects on the sebaceous glands. Surgical removal of the abnormal soft tissue either surgically or by laser usually provides the most satisfactory treatment.

95 i. The diagnosis is borreliosis or Lyme disease. The rash, which may be 'target like' and occurs at the site of tick bites, is known as erythema migrans.
ii. The disease is caused by a spirochaete, *Borrelia burgdorferi*. This is spread by the bite of a tick (a member of the Ixodid family) which has previously bitten and sucked blood from an infected animal (such as a deer). The disease exists thoughout Europe and the USA and varies slightly according to the location.
iii. Borreliosis can also cause an arthritis, cardiac problems (conduction defects in particular), neurological deficits, and skin disorders (acrodermatitis chronica atrophicans and lymphocytoma).
iv. There are serological tests, which are helpful, and biopsy which yields a typical picture with lymphocytes and histiocyes perivascularly. There is also a polymerase chain reaction test, which is quite specific.

96 A 57-year-old male presents with a raised brown–black lesion on his upper back (96). It has irregular pigmentation and irregular margins.
i. What is the most likely diagnosis and what is the main differential diagnosis?
ii. What are the main features of the most likely diagnosis?
iii. What are the main histological features of the most likely diagnosis?

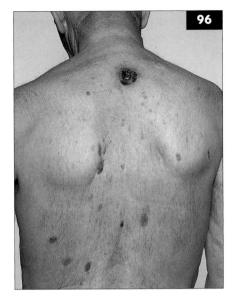

97 An 81-year-old male presents with swollen ankles; he has developed mauve–purple papules and plaques over his toes, feet, and ankles (97). He has been very fit until recently – an Italian by birth, he is convinced that his daily 'dose' of Chianti and liberal helpings of olive oil have kept him in good health.
i. What is the diagnosis?
ii. This disorder may be seen in other clinical settings. What are these?
iii. What treatments are available?
iv. Has there been any recent advance in our understanding of the pathogenesis of this disorder?

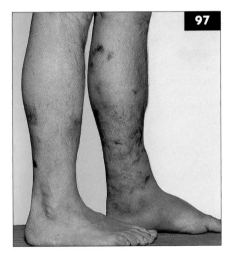

96 i. The most likely clinical diagnosis is nodular malignant melanoma and the main differential diagnosis is seborrhoeic wart.

ii. The main clinical features of malignant melanoma are: enlargement of the lesion over the previous weeks or few months, particularly irregular enlargement; darkening of the pigmentation and variegation (the presence of different shades of brown and black); irregularity of the border of the lesion and of the surface. Late signs include the development of a halo of pigmentation and the presence of pigmented satellite lesions and surface erosion.

iii. The main histological features include extensive proliferation of melanocytic/naevus cells at the dermoepidermal junction. There is increased mitotic activity in these cells, which also show heterogeneity of cell size and shape and nuclear irregularities. They also show upward invasion into the epidermis. Frequently noted additional features are melanin pigment deposits in the upper dermis, both free and within macrophages, and a mixed inflammatory cell infiltrate.

97 i. The disorder is Kaposi's idiopathic haemorrhagic sarcoma. The clinical picture described is the 'classic' form of the disease, which occurs particularly in elderly men who originate from areas of Italy or Russia or who are Ashkenazi Jews. The condition is a multifocal neoplastic disorder of vascular endothelium.

ii. A very aggressive form of the disease occurs in male homosexuals with human immunodeficiency virus (HIV) disease. A similar rapidly progressive form of Kaposi's sarcoma has been described as a rare consequence of immunosuppression in patients who have had renal transplants. In addition, it has been noted to occur in epidemic form in Africa.

iii. Surgery or some form of ablation may be used for isolated lesions but, as the condition is multifocal, is rarely of much assistance. Radiotherapy may help some patients. A topical retinoid has been found to control the disease at the site of application; 0.1% alitretinoin gel (Panretin gel) has been used successfully.

iv. Herpesvirus 8 has been isolated from some Kaposi's lesions.

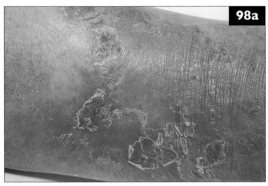

98 A patient presents with a rash that has persisted and spread over a period of 4 months, affecting the groin, neck, face, and axillae (98a). It is oozy and erosive and has not responded to topical treatments.
i. What is the differential diagnosis and what is the most likely diagnosis?
ii. What is the histological characteristic of the most likely diagnosis?
iii. Describe any underlying disorder.

99 A 47-year-old female is experiencing increasing difficulty in opening her mouth wide and in swallowing. She thinks that her face has changed shape and become thinner (99).
i. What is the diagnosis?
ii. Briefly outline the main physical features of this disorder.
iii. What kind of disorder is this?
iv. What is the prognosis?

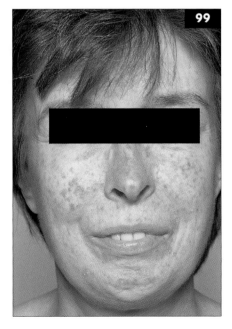

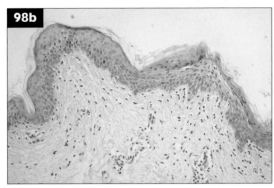

98 i. The differential diagnosis includes seborrhoeic dermatitis, chronic benign familial pemphigus (Hailey–Hailey disease) and necrolytic migratory erythema (NME). NME is the most likely diagnosis as seborrhoeic dermatitis is not usually erosive and usually responds to topical treatment, and Hailey–Hailey disease is a chronic remittent and familial disorder.
ii. The pathognomonic histological feature is a colliquefactive degenerative change in the upper epidermal layers (98b).
iii. NME is usually a sign of a tumour of the pancreatic islet alpha cells – a glucagonoma. Rarely, alpha cell hyperplasia is present rather than a tumour and even more rarely, no underlying pancreatic abnormality can be discovered.

99 i. She has the form of systemic sclerosis known as the CRST syndrome (calcinosis cutis, Raynaud's phenomenon, skin sclerosis and telangiectasia). It is also known as the CREST syndrome – the 'E' standing for oesophageal dysfunction, as this occurs in many patients.
ii. Facial alterations include 'pinched cheeks', microstomia with an overall 'beaked facies' appearance, and macular telangiectasia. The forearms are 'sclerotic' and bound down, as are the fingers, which are also markedly 'tapered' and subject to attacks of Raynaud's phenomenon. Radiographic studies will demonstrate abnormal oesophageal mobility accounting for the dysplasia. In advanced cases small intracutaneous deposits of calcium are found on the hands and fingers.
iii. This disorder is believed to be a type of autoimmune disease and is one variety of systemic sclerosis.
iv. In many patients the disease seems to stabilize but persists. In some less fortunate individuals the disease gradually becomes more extensive and other organ systems are affected (e.g. kidneys, lungs).

100 A female presents because she is concerned about the appearance of her thighs, which are 'lumpy and dimpled' (100). She admits she has put on a bit of weight in recent years.
i. What is the condition of her thighs known as?
ii. What is the disorder due to?
iii. What management should be recommended?

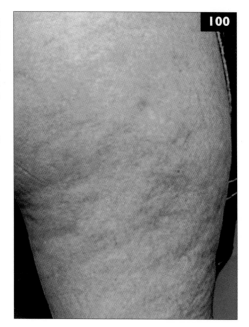

101 A 37-year-old female complains that her fingers go white and cold whenever she exposes her hands to cold water or the cold wind. She also complains that her fingers are becoming stiff and that the skin of her face has also stiffened.
i. The patient clearly has Raynaud's syndrome. What is the likely cause of her Raynaud's disorder?
ii. What other skin signs often accompany the disorder causing her Raynaud's disorder?
iii. What systemic involvements often occur?

102 An 86-year-old female presents with very painful feet. She is otherwise in good health. Examination reveals bilateral bunions with associated callosities, callosities over the dorsa of the metatarsophalangeal joints, and several 'corns' over the soles of the feet.
i. What is the cause of this patient's disablement?
ii. What other conditions may partially imitate this condition?
iii. Briefly describe the management of this condition.

100 i. This is the common condition known as cellulite. Characteristically, it occurs on the front and sides of the thighs of early middle-aged overweight females. It is asymptomatic, but causes much cosmetic distress.

ii. It is thought that the 'lumpy' orange peel appearance is due to a minor gender difference, in that women have subcutaneous fascial compartments that become individually distended with fat tissue.

iii. Despite all the commercial treatments available, only dieting is likely to be successful.

101 i. When the symptoms of Raynaud's syndrome are accompanied by thickening and stiffening of the skin, systemic sclerosis is likely to be the cause of the problem.

ii. The term 'acrosclerosis' is used for the constellation of signs and symptoms seen at the periphery in slowly progressive systemic sclerosis. Apart from the Raynaud's problem, the skin of the hands and forearms is thickened and bound down. In long-standing cases small intracutaneous deposits of calcium around the fingers may be found. Telangiectatic macules may develop over the face.

iii. Systemic sclerosis may involve many systems, but is most commonly a problem of the renal, gastrointestinal, and pulmonary systems.

102 i. This disorder is the result of pain and tenderness caused by the corns, callosities, and bony abnormalities of her feet. These have been caused by the deformities from wearing fashionable rather than comfortable footwear over all her adult life.

ii. Plantar warts (verrucae vulgaris) caused by infection with the human papilloma-virus (antigenic types 1 and 2) are usually found in childhood, adolescence, and young adults. Clinically they are found anywhere over the feet. Their surfaces are studded with pinhead-sized black dots from thrombosed capillaries.

iii. The management involves avoiding further friction with pads and comfortable footwear and reducing the callosities by 'paring' and the use of salicylic acid preparations. Surgical correction of bunions may be needed.

103 A delegation from the World Health Organization was in the middle of a remote Indonesian rainforest and came across a small isolated village. The village was inhabited by a few obviously malnourished people whose bodies and limbs were affected by large crusted sores, 2–5 cm in diameter. They did speak a little English and said that their parents had similar sores, but these had all cleared after the villagers were given an injection.
i. What is the most likely diagnosis? What else could it be?
ii. What is the cause of the most likely diagnosis, and how is it spread? What other disorders are there in this group of diseases?
iii. Does the most likely disorder cause problems in other organ systems?
iv. What is the treatment of this disorder?

104 On Monday, after working hard in the garden over the hot weekend, a male presents with itchy red streaks on his chest, forearms, and face (104).
i. What is the most likely diagnosis?
ii. Describe the pathogenesis of this condition.
iii. How should this disorder be managed?

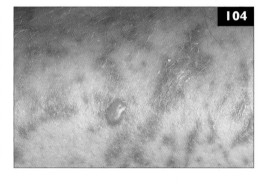

105 A 38-year-old female noticed the mask-like symmetrical brown discolouration of the skin of her face in the previous 8 months (105). It seems to fluctuate in intensity, but is tending to gradually worsen.
i. What is the differential diagnosis?
ii. Outline the aetiology.
iii. Outline the management.

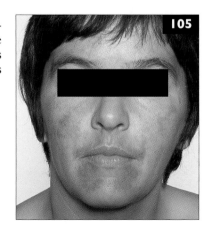

103 i. The most likely diagnosis is yaws. Another possibility is ecthyma, although lesions in this disorder tend to be erosive rather than crusted. Lesions of Buruli ulcer are usually larger and few in number.

ii. Yaws is caused by *Treponema pertenue*. It occurs in impoverished and isolated communities and is spread by direct contact. The other members of the treponematoses group are pinta, infectious syphilis, and venereal syphilis. The *Treponema* sp. responsible for yaws is virtually identical with *T. pallidum*, which causes syphilis.

iii. Yaws can cause an arthropathy, a periostitis, and malaise. It can also cause destruction of the nasal mucosa and destruction of the nasal bridge in the late stages, just as in syphilis. It can also cause various ophthalmological complications.

iv. The treatment is straightforward and usually successful – one injection of benzathine penicillin is sufficient. The whole community should be treated together.

104 i. The most likely diagnosis is phytophotodermatitis.

ii. The condition is basically an acute eczema resulting from a combination of being splashed and squirted with the sap of certain common plants, such as cow parsley, which contains photosensitizing coumarins, and exposure to the sun.

iii. Usually the condition settles within a few days and is improved symptomatically by the use of topical corticosteroids. Clearly the cause of the condition needs to be explained to the patient so that he does not risk having a recurrence.

105 i. The light brown discolouration occurring symmetrically on the forehead, cheeks, and temples is typical of melasma (chloasma). It occurs predominantly in women in the reproductive years, but is occasionally seen in men. It has to be distinguished from pigmentation due to Addison's disease, which is more marked in flexures and occurs on skin elsewhere. It must also be differentiated from the pigmentation due to certain drugs (e.g. minocycline) and disturbances of pigmentation due to the yeast infection pityriasis versicolor.

ii. Little is known of the cause of this disorder, other than it is seen in pregnancy and after some oral contraceptives.

iii. A combination of hydroquinone, tretinoin, and potent topical steroids are used in the USA, but this is not licensed in the UK (for other countries see individual regulations). Topical azelaic acid (20%) is quite effective in some patients after 2–3 months of use. Sun tan accentuates the problem and affected individuals need to use effective sun protection.

106 Several children in the same school have developed the condition seen in 106.
i. What is this disorder? What clinical features are common in this condition?
ii. What is the cause of this disease?
iii. What treatment should be recommended?

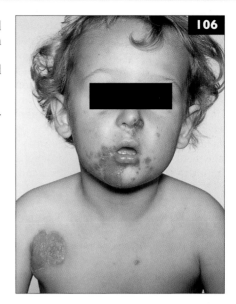

107 A 74-year-old female was injured by a supermarket trolley on her left ankle about 3 months ago and the area has not healed despite her best efforts (107).
i. What is the most likely diagnosis and what other diagnoses should be considered?
ii. What is the aetiopathogenesis of the most likely diagnosis?
iii. What management should be recommended?

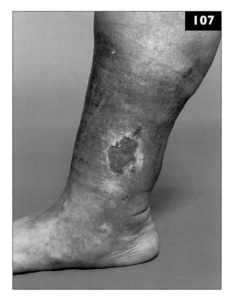

106 i. This disorder is impetigo contagiosa. Pink, scaling, slightly thickened patches appear, which become oozy and develop a golden yellow crust. While patches often develop on the face, they can occur anywhere and it is common to have more than one.

ii. The cause of the disorder is infection of the skin with *Staphylococcus aureus* or beta-haemolytic *Streptococcus* after direct contact with a lesion on another infected individual. There appear to be geographic differences in the bacteriological cause.

iii. Treatment may be topical or by the oral systemic route. Topically, the antibiotics fucidin, neomycin, or mupirocin may be used alongside detergent antimicrobial agents to wash affected sites. Systemically, penicillin V is still a very suitable drug, although semi-synthetic penicillins and fluoroquinolones are also useful.

107 i. The most likely diagnosis is a venous ulcer. These are usually located just above the medial malleolus, but often spread around the ankle circumferentially. The ankle may be slightly swollen and the skin of the ankle around the ulcer is often irregularly pigmented and there are many visibly dilated blood vessels in the subcutis (the appearance being known as a venous flare). Other diagnoses that should be considered include ischaemia, squamous cell carcinoma, and diabetic ulceration.

ii. The deep long veins of the lower legs and communicating perforating veins become incompetent because of disordered function of the venous valves. Venous blood is normally returned to the heart by the pumping action of the calf muscles and the prevention of retrograde flow by the venous valves. The result of the incompetence of the valves is increased venous pressure in the veins (venous hypertension). This leads to oedema, fibrin deposition, hypoxaemia, and eventually ulceration.

iii. Management should be directed to improving the venous drainage by support bandaging (with either crepe bandage or elasticated stockings), weight reduction, daily leg elevation, and gentle exercise of the calf muscles. The ulcerated surface should be protected from the environment with a nonadherent dressing possessing an antimicrobial surface.

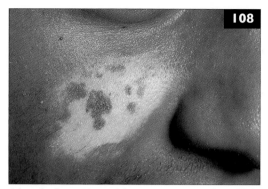

108 An 11-year-old male from West Africa presents with well-defined white areas on the backs of his hands and elsewhere over the skin surface (108).
i. Discuss the differential diagnosis.
ii. Describe the pathogenesis and pathology of the most likely diagnosis.
iii. What is the prognosis and what is the most appropriate management?

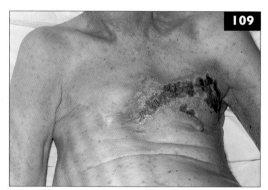

109 i. What is this male suffering from (109)?
ii. Briefly discuss the cause.
iii. Briefly discuss associations and complications of this disorder.

108 i. The occurrence of hypopigmented areas in someone with pigmented skin is always a cause of concern. If the areas are well defined and symmetrical, vitiligo is the most frequent cause. In a country in which leprosy is endemic the presence of hypopigmented macules must be regarded with suspicion. Hypoaesthesia and the presence of enlarged peripheral nerves support the diagnosis of leprosy. Pityriasis versicolor is nearly always slightly scaly and occurs in a confetti-like distribution mainly over the upper trunk. Examination of skin scrapings for *Pityrosporon ovale* (*Malassezia furfur*), skin snips for leprosy bacillus, and skin biopsies to support a diagnosis of vitiligo may assist in confirming the clinical diagnosis.

ii. The most likely diagnosis is vitiligo which is thought to belong to the organ-specific group of autoimmune diseases. Pigment-producing cells (melanocytes) are evident normally as clear cells along the basal layer of the epidermis (approximately 5% of the basal cells), but have disappeared in the hypopigmented areas of vitiligo. It is thought that they are targeted by cytotoxic T-lymphocytes, although the antigen responsible and the triggering mechanism are uncertain. There is a familial predisposition with a HLA susceptibility.

iii. The prognosis for vitiligo is uncertain. In some cases there is spontaneous remission, but in most instances the depigmented areas spread slowly but relentlessly. Some improvement has been claimed for treatment by photochemo-therapy with ultraviolet A (PUVA). Improvement has also been claimed for topical treatment with corticosteroids and pimecrolimus as well as systemic immuno-modulatory drugs. For the most part, and certainly in most lightly pigmented individuals, treatment may be restricted to camouflage with stains such as 2% dihydroxyacetone.

109 i. The disorder is herpes zoster, also known as shingles.

ii. The cause of herpes zoster is the reactivation of the varicella-zoster virus in the appropriate posterior root ganglion and its migration along the posterior (sensory) root to the skin. The zoster virus is a small DNA virus of the herpes group. The condition only occurs in people who have had varicella (chicken pox) in the past. Reactivation of the virus and zoster mostly occurs in the elderly for no apparent reason. However, it also develops when there is a reduction in the immune defences as in patients with human immunodeficiency virus (HIV) disease or who are on immunosuppressant drugs.

iii. Herpes zoster can be very painful. It is also the cause of persistent odd paraesthesiae in the area of the skin innervated by the affected nerve. Long-standing burning pain in the affected area is a problem in 20–30% of patients.

110 The skin condition in **110** is on the lower leg of a 52-year-old man who complains bitterly of itch.
i. What is the most likely diagnosis and what is the differential diagnosis?
ii. What are the main histological features?
iii. What is the treatment and prognosis?

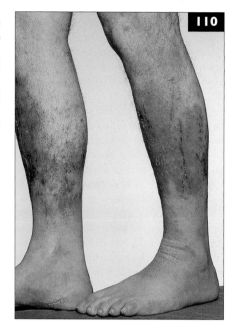

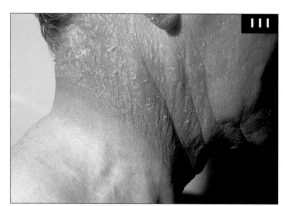

111 A gardener, aged 64, presents with a rash that has developed over the past 3 months and which seems to get worse each time he works outdoors (**111**).
i. What is the likely diagnosis?
ii. Describe important physical features of this condition.
iii. Discuss the management of the disorder.

110 i. The persistent severe itching and the well-defined, thickened warty and/or scaling red patch are typical of lichen simplex chronicus (also known as circumscribed neurodermatitis). The condition may be solitary or there may be several such patches. Psoriasis may look similar, but is not usually very itchy. Hypertrophic lichen planus may be quite similar in appearance, although is often more mauve in colour.

ii. Regular and sometimes massive epidermal thickening without the inflammatory components of psoriasis characterize the condition histologically.

iii. Potent topical corticosteroids and tar preparations form the basis of treatment, but regrettably are not very effective. Occlusive dressings with potent topical corticosteroid preparations are sometimes helpful. The condition usually remits spontaneously after several months.

111 i. The likely diagnosis is chronic actinic dermatitis.

ii. The eruption is worse on the most exposed sites of the forehead, cheeks, ears, and back of the neck, but the upper lip and upper eyelids are relatively spared. There may also be a dyspigmentation in patients who have had the disorder some time.

iii. Patients will require testing to determine to which wavelengths they are sensitive; such testing is performed by use of a monochromator in specialized photobiology units. In addition, the patients should be patch tested and also tested by photo patch testing to determine the presence of both allergic contact hypersensitivities and photosensitivities. The most important aspect of their management is the avoidance of exposure of their skin to the ultraviolet radiation (UVR) wavelengths responsible for the problem. Patients are sometimes exquisitely sensitive to UVR and they must be careful to block all sources of UVR. Sunscreens rarely have the ability to block all the responsible wavelengths, but should nonetheless be used to reduce the dose received. The rash itself may be treated with topical steroids and emollients, but often more powerful systemic agents such as azathioprine and ciclosporin may need to be used.

112 i. What is the cause of this patient's nail problem (**112**)? He says that he did have an itchy red rash affecting the wrists, arms, and legs, but this disappeared after about 6 months.
ii. What other sites are sometimes affected in this disorder?
iii. Discuss the management of this condition.

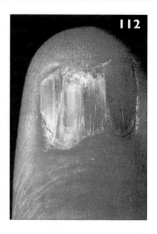

113 A 6-year-old boy is brought to the clinic by his mother who has noticed small irregular pale areas of skin on his cheeks, neck, and both upperarms in the past 4 weeks. They are increasing in number and seem to have a slight scale on their surface.
i. Briefly discuss the differential diagnosis.
ii. In what type of patient and at what body site does the most likely diagnosis occur?
iii. Outline the management of this case.

114 A 70-year-old male presents with painful red spots that recurrently affect the chest and back (**114**).
i. What is the most likely diagnosis?
ii. Are there many precipitating or aggravating factors that could be relevant in this case?
iii. What management should be recommended?

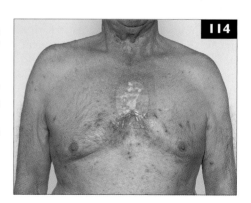

112 i. The nail in the photograph belongs to a patient with lichen planus. The linear ridging is typical. When severe the condition can cause permanent destruction of the nail.

ii. Lichen planus frequently affects the buccal mucosa (an estimated 25–30%). It less commonly affects other mucosal sites such as the vagina. It may also affect the scalp, where it produces areas of alopecia with scarring.

iii. Lichen planus has a prominent immunopathological component and immuno-suppressive agents can suppress the disease, notably steroids and ciclosporin. However, the involvement of the nails is very difficult to improve and when nail destruction with scarring occurs nothing can be done. The disease usually goes into remission at some unpredictable point after months or years.

113 i. The parents are most concerned as to the possibility of leprosy as they have emigrated from an area where leprosy is endemic. The symmetrical distribution and the slight surface scale make leprosy unlikely and the diagnosis of pityriasis simplex, an eczematous disorder, is much more likely. The possibilities of vitiligo and pityriasis versicolor must also be considered. The depigmentation in vitiligo is much more profound and pityriasis versicolor is generally a disorder of adolescents and young adults.

ii. For the most part, pityriasis simplex occurs in children aged 2–8 years and in those with a pigmented skin or at least a dark complexion.

iii. The diagnosis should be established, if necessary using skin snips to exclude leprosy, and skin scrapings to detect the presence of spores and the pseudomycelium of pityriasis versicolor. A full-thickness skin biopsy is rarely needed, but should be considered if there is still doubt. Once pityriasis simplex is confirmed, emollients and diluted corticosteroids may be used. The condition tends to remit spontaneously after some months.

114 i. The most likely diagnosis is 'late-onset acne'. This is more common than was once thought and, with the recent change in the national demographic profile, a larger number of elderly patients with acne is seen now than was once the case. Truncal acne in elderly men is a frequent presentation.

ii. Drugs of various kinds can precipitate and/or aggravate the condition including corticosteroids and anabolic steroids. Working in prolonged humidity can also be responsible.

iii. Management is much the same as for younger patients, but particular care needs to be taken to search for precipitating/aggravating factors. Prolonged courses of low-dose oral isotretinoin have been successfully used.

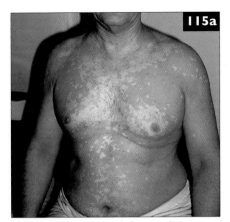

115 i. What is the differential diagnosis of the condition seen in 115a?
ii. What are the most typical clinical features of the most likely diagnosis?
iii. Briefly discuss the prognosis and treatment.

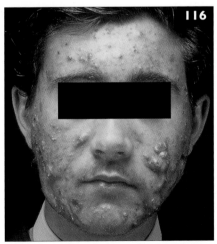

116 A 23-year-old male has had facial acne for several years that has failed to respond to topical agents or to systemic antibiotics. In the last 2 or 3 weeks the condition seemed to suddenly worsen, with many more lesions developing and worsening of the pre-existing papules and cysts (116).
i. What is a possible explanation for the worsening?
ii. Are there any systematic accompaniments to the patient's problem?
iii. What treatment should be recommended?

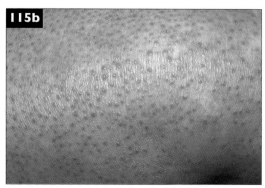

115 i. The involvement of face and scalp with red scaling plaques and spread to trunk and limbs is typical of pityriasis rubra pilaris (PRP). The lesions tend to be 'psoriasiform' and alternative diagnoses are psoriasis and chronic eczema.
ii. In some sites the follicles contain horny plugs or spines (115b). The rash often has an 'orangey hue'. Uninvolved white islands are also evident.
iii. Most patients with PRP are clear after 18 months to 2 years, but are subject to recurrences. Topical agents may provide a degree of symptomatic relief. Methotrexate and azathioprine give some assistance. Ciclosporin does not help. The oral retinoids are the most effective treatment for PRP, but patients may not consider the side-effects worth the improvement in their disease.

116 i. It seems that the patient's acne has progressed to the condition of acne fulminans or pyoderma faciale. There is no adequate explanation for this sudden aggravation, although it has been suggested that some immunological event is responsible. It has also been suggested that pyoderma faciale is in fact a different condition from acne fulminans and is in reality a form of rosacea. However, there is no evidence in favour of this concept.
ii. Patients with acne fulminans feel ill and often have a low pyrexia. A leukaemoid level of leucocytosis may be noted. In addition, patients may experience joint pain and on radiographs small cyst-like translucent areas may be seen at the ends of long bones. Splenomegaly is also a feature in some patients.
iii. Antibiotics, such as the tetracyclines or erythromycin in full dosage, and systemic steroids are usually administered. Isotretinoin is also usually prescribed, carefully matching dose to side-effects. Dapsone is also given depending on the progress.

117 An 83-year-old male was admitted to hospital for a flare of his chronic obstructive pulmonary disease (COPD). After 1 week he complains of some itchiness on his lower legs (117).
i. What is this condition?
ii. What is the cause?
iii. How should it be treated?

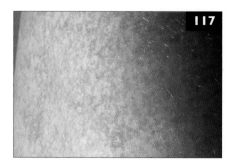

118 A male aged 27 presents with brown–grey patches that have developed on his face in the past 6 months. He also has quite noticeable acne and together they constitute a real cosmetic problem.
i. What is the most likely cause of his pigmentary problem?
ii. Are there any other possible adverse side-effects that may be due to the causative agent?
iii. What management should be recommended?

119 A female presents with swelling of the neck that has developed over the last 9 months. Her husband has noticed that she has become 'jumpy' and that her eyes seem brighter and more prominent than they used to be. A circumscribed pink thickened patch has developed over the right shin (119) in the past 3 or 4 months and there is a hint of the same problem starting on the left shin.
i. What is the most likely diagnosis?
ii. What other signs of skin involvement may develop in this condition?
iii. Briefly discuss the pathogenesis of this condition.

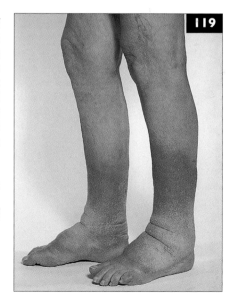

117 i. The disorder is known as eczema cracquelée or asteatotic eczema.

ii. It results from a combination of overzealous rubbing and scrubbing by the nursing staff and low relative humidity in an elderly individual who is generally unwell.

iii. It should be treated by a reduction in vigorous toilet procedures and by the regular use of emollients.

118 i. The most likely explanation for the pigmentary problem is that the patient has been taking minocycline for his acne and that he has developed the pigmentation occasionally seen due to this drug. The exact chemistry is uncertain, but it appears that minocycline and/or its metabolites form insoluble complexes that become fixed in superficial tissues of skin. Pigmentation may occur in light-exposed sites, in scars, or at the periphery of the limbs.

ii. Other adverse side-effects of minocycline include a systemic lupus erythematosus (SLE)-like syndrome in which a rheumatoid arthritis-like picture, a hepatitis, and a pneumonitis all may occur. Minocycline may also cause a fixed drug eruption.

iii. There are no specific means of accelerating the removal of the pigment; it does, however, gradually disappear.

119 i. The most likely diagnosis is hyperthyroidism (Grave's disease) and pretibial myxoedema.

ii. The site of predilection is the shin and it has been surmised that this is because the shin is prone to minor injury. It is usual for the contralateral shin to also be involved, although this may only be to a minor degree. Involvement of the dorsa of the hands and the fingers is also quite common. When the fingers are affected the finger tips are sometimes clubbed and the condition is then known as thyroid acropachy.

iii. The condition is thought to be autoimmune in origin, the thyroid-simulating hormone receptor possibly being the pivotal target. The condition is strongly associated with exophthalmos and ophthalmoplegia. There is usually elevated serum long-acting thyroid stimulator, and it has been found that serum from affected patients stimulates fibroblasts *in vitro* to secrete hyaluronic acid.

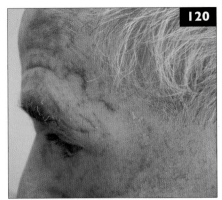

120 An 88-year-old retired miner presents with bluish marks on his forehead (120) and on the dorsa of his hands.
i. What is the most likely explanation for these and what is the differential diagnosis?
ii. Name some other stigmata analogous to the most likely diagnosis in this case.
iii. What is the most appropriate form of management?

121 A male has psoriasis that has become generalized in the past 3 months despite being on methotrexate. He has had several courses of photochemotherapy with ultraviolet A (PUVA) previously and the PUVA with acitretin that he has been given on this occasion has not helped. Briefly discuss each of the following possibilities of management.
i. Start intensive topical treatment as an inpatient and if necessary add oral weekly methotrexate.
ii. Start ciclosporin treatment.
iii. Start treatment with an anti-tumour necrosis factor alpha (TNF-α) agent, one of the biologics (e.g. etanercept, infliximab).

122 A teenager, who is keen on sport, complains that he came out in an itchy rash after playing squash.
i. What is this disorder?
ii. When else might it be seen?
iii. Does it differ much from similar rashes caused by other stimuli?
iv. What treatment should be advised?

120 i. The bluish marks are most likely to be due to minor injury against jutting-out coal seams, with consequent tattooing. Such marks were at one time common amongst miners, but since the decline of coal mining are now rarely seen. Attempts at tattooing and subsequent removal may produce similar marks. Blue naevi could be confused with 'coal marks'.

ii. Agricultural workers often have thick callosities from handling farm implements; violinists often have thickened ruggose skin on the side of the neck; boxers and rugby players have thickened and misshapen ears (cauliflower ears).

iii. The most appropriate form of management is reassurance alone. Apart from overtattooing with a lighter colour, there is no other available treatment.

121 i. Intensive topical treatment is facilitated by inpatient treatment or by supervision in a day treatment centre; it is difficult to find the necessary facilities. In addition, such treatment is mostly unpopular with patients and is slow to take effect.

ii. Ciclosporin treatment is rapidly effective, but has serious toxicities curtailing treatment: hypertension and nephrotoxicities as well as predisposing to infection and neoplastic disease.

iii. The 'biologics' include etanercept, infliximab, and adalimumab. They are given systemically and are quite effective, but unfortunately are quite expensive. With etanercept 48% of patients achieved 75% reduction in psoriasis area severity index (PASI) score at 12 weeks with 50 mg twice weekly. Infliximab is similarly effective. Benefits of combining the biologics with other systemic agents have been demonstrated.

122 i. The disorder is cholinergic urticaria.

ii. It is seen after any form of strenuous exercise and after hot baths.

iii. The individual urticarial lesions are small papules, rather than the variably sized but larger hives seen in other urticarial conditions. Patchy macular erythema may also occur, as may systemic symptoms.

iv. The condition responds poorly to antihistamines. Anticholinergic drugs sometimes help.

123 An 83-year-old female presents with a painful foot and the condition on the front of her shins and knees is noticed incidentally (123). She lives by herself in a cottage with no central heating. To keep warm she has to sit right in front of her open fire.
i. What is this condition?
ii. What is it due to?
iii. Does this condition have any complications?

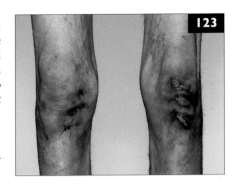

124 A 24-year-old female presents, feeling unwell. She is losing some scalp hair and complains of pains in her wrists, ankles, and hands. She has also developed a red rash across her face (124).
i. What is the differential diagnosis and what is the most likely diagnosis?
ii. What laboratory test findings might be expected in the most likely diagnosis?
iii. What other systems may be affected in the most likely diagnosis?

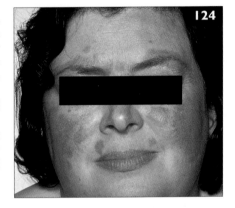

125 A 50-year-old female presents with a generalized itch she has had for the past 4 years (125).
i. Which skin diseases may present with pruritus, but eventuate into visible skin disorders?
ii. What investigations are needed in this patient?
iii. If all the investigations fail to reveal an abnormality, what is your most likely diagnosis.

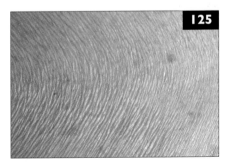

105

123 i. The condition is erythema ab igne. Characteristically, there is a persistent red–brown network over the affected skin. Small warty areas and ulcers may also develop subsequently in the affected area.

ii. It is a type of chronic heat injury and is found in other body sites subjected to long continued or intermittent heating (e.g. on the back or abdomen if constantly warmed by a hot water bottle).

iii. The heat injury may occasionally cause premalignant lesions: keratoses and even squamous cell carcinoma.

124 i. The list of differential diagnoses includes systemic lupus erythematosus (SLE), rosacea, dermatomyositis, seborrhoeic dermatitis, and the carcinoid syndrome. SLE is the most likely diagnosis given the general disorder the patient has. The lack of inflammatory papules, scaling, flushing, or muscular pain and tenderness rules out some of the other possibilities and increases the likelihood of SLE.

ii. All cellular elements of blood including thrombocytes may be deficient. The antinuclear factor test is positive as is the test for antibodies to double-stranded DNA. Abnormalities in immunoglobulins and complement levels are also often present.

iii. Hepatosplenomegaly may be present. Lupus nephritis, lupoid hepatitis, meningoencephalitis, and lupoid pneumonitis are other serious systemic complications.

125 i. Senile pemphigoid occasionally first presents as generalized pruritus without much of a rash. The same is true of the itchy blistering condition dermatitis herpetiformis.

ii. Chronic renal failure, hyperparathyroidism, hyperthyroidism, biliary obstruction, and lymphoma may all cause generalized pruritus. The appropriate blood tests need to be performed to exclude these possibilities.

iii. Many patients with generalized pruritus seem fit in all other aspects. All that can be observed on the skin are the results of scratching – excoriations and prurigo papules. Some of these patients are elderly and have a 'dryish' skin. For these the label senile xerosis is used. For the others the terms idiopathic pruritus and neurotic excoriations are unsatisfactory but are nonetheless frequently used.

126 A male presents with a generalized rash that consists of numerous pink maculopapular elements (**126**). It is nonitchy and also affects the palms. It has been present for the past 2 weeks. He feels generally unwell and on examination he is found to have a degree of lymph node enlargement in the neck, axillae, and groins. There are also shallow erosions in the mouth.

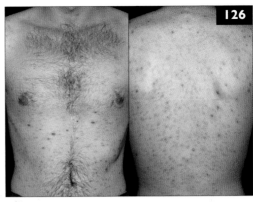

i. What diagnosis must be considered?
ii. Are there particular questions that need to be answered?
iii. What is the most appropriate treatment for the most likely diagnosis?

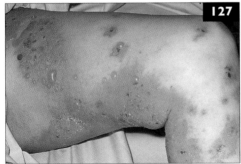

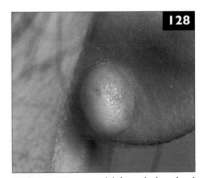

127 i. What is the most likely disorder to account for the blistering shown in **127**? What kind of person may develop this condition?
ii. Describe the characteristic features of the disease.
iii. Briefly describe the histological features.
iv. What are the main immunological findings.

128 An 18-year-old female has had lumps on her ear lobes (**128**) for the past 4 months.
i. What is the differential diagnosis?
ii. What is the most likely diagnosis and how would this be confirmed?
iii. What is the recommended management of the most likely diagnosis?

126 i. A strong possibility is that the diagnosis is secondary syphilis. The exanthematic stage of human immunodeficiency virus (HIV) disease can also demonstrate very similar features but shows less in the way of mucosal lesions and lymphadenopathy. The exanthem of glandular fever may also show a similar set of physical signs.

ii. A detailed history of recent sexual contacts is important. Itching should be specifically enquired about as the rash of secondary syphilis is generally nonpruritic.

iii. It is vital to be certain about the diagnosis, therefore blood should taken for serological tests for syphilis, tests for HIV, and tests for infectious mononucleosis. If necessary, skin biopsy should be performed. When the diagnosis of secondary syphilis is certain, a 2-week treatment with systemic penicillin (2 mega units daily), is administered.

127 i. Senile bullous pemphigoid. The condition is seen in the elderly. It does not appear to be more common in those with underlying neoplastic disease, as was once thought.

ii. Often considerable itching accompanies the disease. The blisters arise on normal-appearing skin and are tense and usually contain some blood-stained fluid. They may arise anywhere on the skin, but do not usually involve the oral mucosa.

iii. The blisters arise subepidermally. The inflammatory cell infiltrate may contain many eosinophils.

iv. The main immunological features include circulating IgG antibodies directed against epidermal hemidesmosomal proteins of 180KD and 230KD. The titre of the antibodies approximately parallels the disease activity. Direct immuno-fluorescence tests on skin biopsy material demonstrate the presence of IgG and C3 complement component in the skin around the blistered area.

128 i. The differential diagnosis includes ear piercing keloid scars, granuloma from ear piercing, and cutaneous sarcoidosis.

ii. The most likely diagnosis is ear piercing keloid scars. Clearly the patient must be asked if she (or he) has had ear piercing. Biopsy will reveal the typical histological picture of keloid scar.

iii. Intralesional injection of a corticosteriod may help some patients. The lesions can be excised, but as with keloids at other sites there is a danger of recurrence.

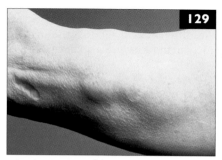

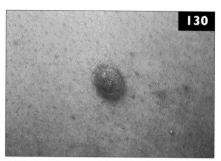

129 A 37-year-old male presents with a series of soft swellings on his arms and trunk (129). They started some 5 years ago and are slowly increasing in size and number. Some of these lesions are occasionally painful.
i. What are these lesions and what is the differential diagnosis?
ii. What would a biopsy reveal?
iii. What management should be recommended?

130 A 12-year-old male has had this orange–pink dome-shaped lesion (130) on his arm for the past 8 months.
i. What is the most likely diagnosis?
ii. What differential diagnosis ought to be considered?
iii. What may the histological picture be mistaken for? Describe the main histological feature of the most likely diagnosis.

131 A female patient reports that her legs didn't look 'the same'. One leg seems thinner and pinker than the other (131).
i. What is a possible explanation for this?
ii. Are there other cutaneous side-effects from the use of topical treatment that might be present?
iii. Are there systemic side-effects that might also develop from the use of this topical medication?

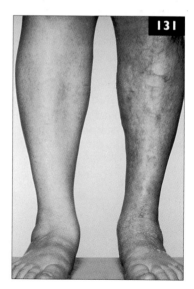

129 i. These are almost certainly lipomata – benign tumours of adipose tissue. Neurofibroma should be considered in the differential diagnosis although, if multiple, would be part of Von Recklinghausen's disease, which also demonstrates *café au lait* patches on the skin.
ii. A biopsy would reveal normal-looking fat tissue only.
iii. The only management required is reassurance as to the benign nature of the disorder and removal of any lesion that is mechanically or cosmetically disabling and is surgically feasible.

130 i. The most likely diagnosis is juvenile melanoma (Spitz naevus). The red, *peau d' orange* surface is characteristic.
ii. The list of differential diagnoses includes angioma, compound naevus, and juvenile xanthogranuloma.
iii. The histological appearance can be misinterpreted as a malignant melanoma. The main features are the presence of abundant junctional collections of large mole cells, large strap-like mole cells, and many giant cells, and an epidermal reaction characterized by exaggeration of the rete pattern.

131 i. The most likely explanation is that the patient has been applying a potent topical corticosteriod for a long time and the changes observed are due to profound skin atrophy. This particular patient had used fluocinonide 0.05% over a 6-year period. She was originally prescribed the cream for a patch of eczema and she continued to obtain the preparation on repeat prescription and use it to suppress the irritation.
ii. Other cutaneous side-effects from the use of topical corticosteroids include striae distensae and difficult to recognize (or 'disguised') ringworm infection (tinea incognito).
iii. Systemic side-effects develop when significant amounts of topical corticosteroids are used and the contained corticosteroids are absorbed. Pituitary adrenal axis suppression occurs when sufficient steroid is absorbed through the skin. If 70 g, or more, of 0.1% betamethasone-17-valerate cream or ointment or 30 g, or more, of clobetasol-17-propionate are used per week, sufficient is absorbed to suppress the pituitary adrenal axis. This can lead to an adrenal crisis and collapse. Iatrogenic Cushing's syndrome develops when large amounts of the corticosteroid are absorbed from the topical preparation over long periods.

132 A 60-year-old male patient has several lesions on his arms and legs (**132**).
i. What is the most likely diagnosis and what are the main differential diagnoses?
ii. What investigations may help in establishing the diagnosis?
iii. Outline the management of this patient.

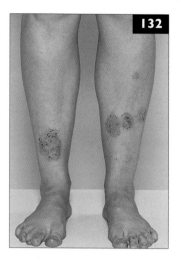

133 A 43-year-old male has developed a reddish-brown plaque over his nose and adjoining right cheek over the past 6 months.
i. What diagnoses should be considered and which of these is the most likely?
ii. What is the characteristic histological appearance of the most likely diagnosis?
iii. What treatments have been found helpful for this condition?

134 A 27-year-old female complains that her skin, which has always felt rough, is worsening, particularly over her arms and thighs (**134**).
i. What is this disorder?
ii. Describe the main clinical features.
iii. Is the disorder associated with any other diseases?

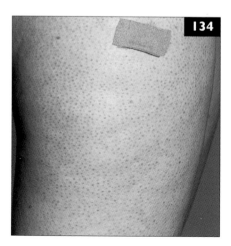

111

132 i. The most likely diagnosis of a disc- or coin-shaped red scaling lesion on the arms and/or legs is discoid eczema. Other diagnoses that need to be considered include ringworm (often ring shaped) and psoriasis (evidence of the disease previously and elsewhere such as elbows, knees, and scalp is helpful).
ii. Examination of skin scales after clearing in 20% potassium hydroxide will reveal fragments of hyphae (mycelium) in ringworm. A punch biopsy should distinguish discoid eczema from psoriasis because of the regular epidermal hyperplasia in the latter. It will also clearly differentiate Bowen's disease and superficial basal cell carcinoma, which may sometimes have a similar clinical appearance.
iii. Having established the diagnosis the treatment should be with moderately potent or potent topical corticosteroids. It is customary to also prescribe an emollient as there is often an accompanying mild xeroderma.

133 i. Sarcoidosis, discoid lupus erythematosus, or a mycobacterial infection should be considered, but the most likely diagnosis is granuloma faciale, which appears to be a type of vasculitis with similarities to erythema elevatum diutinum. It mostly develops in men and is virtually restricted to the face.
ii. Characteristically, there is a moderately dense mixed inflammatory cell infiltrate with lymphocytes, polymorphonuclear leucocytes (as well as polymorphonuclear cell debris), and eosinophils in the upper and mid dermis around the micro-vasculature, which may also show endothelial cell swelling and fibrin deposition.
iii. Intralesional steroid has been reported as helpful, but recently, laser treatment has been found to be a genuine advance in efficacy. Success has also been claimed with topical pimecrolimus 1%.

134 i. This disorder is keratosis pilaris. Uncommon variants include keratosis pilaris rubra, in which there is perifollicular redness, and keratosis pilaris atrophicans (also known as ulerythema ophryogenes).
ii. This common disorder of children and adolescents is characterized by roughened areas of skin on the upper arms and thighs in which the follicles are filled by horny plugs.
iii. Keratosis pilaris is associated with autosomal dominant ichthyosis and atopic dermatitis.

135 An 18-year-old male, who is otherwise quite fit, suddenly developed a papular rash 6 weeks ago. Some of the lesions were crusted and a few actually blistered (135) which made his parents think of chicken pox. As he had contracted chicken pox as a child and the present rash has persisted, it is clearly not that.
i. What it the likely diagnosis?
ii. Describe the pathology of the most likely diagnosis.
iii. Discuss the prognosis and the management of the most likely diagnosis.

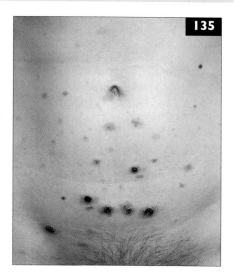

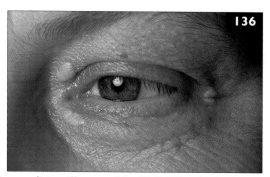

136 i. What is the condition illustrated in 136? What is the basis of the disorder?
ii. In what conditions does this disorder occur?
iii. How should this disorder be treated?

137 A patient presents with itchy lumps on the skin, which are induced by exposure to the cold. This is a particular problem when going swimming.
i. What is the diagnosis?
ii. What investigations are worthwhile?
iii. What other physical stimuli can induce a similar response?

135 i. The most likely diagnosis is that of pityriasis lichenoides et varioliformis acuta (PLEVA). Uncommonly, multiple insect bites can look a little like PLEVA but these are usually surmounted by a punctum and there may be an associated blood crust. Furthermore the lesions of PLEVA are distributed predominantly on the trunk as opposed to insect bites which tend to be on the limbs.
ii. The pathological changes are mainly in the upper dermis and epidermis. Typically, the epidermis is permeated by monocytes and there is an inflammatory cell infiltrate in the upper dermis containing monocytes. In a few patients some of these cells may appear atypical. There may be apoptotic cells scattered in the epidermis, and epidermal necrosis in the most severe cases. There is often a parakeratotic crust.
iii. The condition is remittent, but may persist for several months or even years. The condition does not respond to any topical treatment and does not usually respond to systemic therapies, although tetracyclines have been claimed to help. However, PLEVA does respond to treatment with ultraviolet radiation with ultraviolet B.

136 i. The condition is xanthelasma. It is the result of deposition of lipid in histiocytes in the upper dermis.
ii. In most subjects with this condition there is no systemic abnormality. In some 20% there is hyperlipidaemia of some type.
iii. In those with hyperlipidaemia appropriate treatment with diet and lipid-lowering agents is necessary. If there is no obvious systemic disorder, treatment by surgery may be performed. An alternative is to carefully blanche the affected area by dabbing the yellow plaques with trichloracetic acid.

137 i. This is cold urticaria. It is sometimes associated with cryoglobulinaemia, paraproteinaemia, and autoimmune disorders.
ii. Confirmation can be obtained by placing an ice block on the skin surface (**137**). Examination of the blood for cryoproteins is required.
iii. Solar exposure, pressure, and water can all induce a similar urticarial response in a few patients.

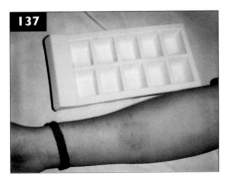

138 A 15-year-old male presents with 'stretch marks' over the middle of the back (138), the upper arms, and thighs that cause him some distress.
i. What is the cause of the stretch marks?
ii. What is their treatment?
iii. What is the long-term outlook?

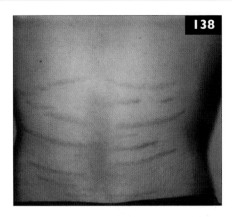

139 A 78-year-old male presents with an increasing number of warty lesions on his scalp (139). He had been a merchant seaman and a building labourer. He had started to lose his hair at the age of 40.
i. What is the most likely diagnosis?
ii. Briefly discuss the treatment options.
iii. How could these lesions have been prevented?

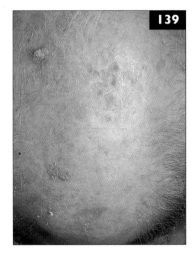

140 A male presents with a rash, which is preceded by discomfort and burning; only the parts of the skin exposed to the sun were affected. The rash itself consists of urticarial weals and a degree of swelling and is quite itchy. The patient sometimes feels nauseated when the rash is present. Being in the sun for just a few moments is enough to provoke the rash.
i. What is the diagnosis and the differential diagnosis?
ii. What is the most likely inciting wavelength?
iii. Discuss the management.

138 i. The cause of the stretch marks (striae distensae) is an increase in intra-cutaneous mechanical strains and a comparative weakening of the dermal connec-tive tissue resulting in the rupture of elastic fibres. Striae are seen in normal physiological states such as the adolescent growth spurt and pregnancy when there is excess glucocorticoid activity. Striae are also seen in both therapeutic and pathological hypercortisonism. They also arise as a result of treatment with systemic corticosteroids or from the administration of corticosteroids locally, especially the very potent topical steroids.
ii. There is no effective treatment, although many drugs, including topical retinoids, have been advocated.
iii. Striae distensae start off purple or deep red and after some months become pale until eventually they become white and seem to shrink (striae albicantes).

139 i. The most likely diagnosis is multiple solar keratoses.
ii. The treatment will depend on the number, size, and sites of the lesions, as well as the general health and well-being of the patient. When there are only a few lesions present, curettage and cautery is safe and effective. Cryotherapy has been popular with dermatologists (but not their patients!), but it is not always effective and is always painful. Treatment with 5% fluorouracil, 3% diclofenac, or 5% imiquimod are alternative topical treatments that are particularly appropriate for multiple lesions in frail patients. Photodynamic therapy using a porphyrin derivative and a beam of light is a promising new form of treatment in which dysplastic tissue is selectively killed.
iii. Reduction in solar exposure reduces the likelihood of solar keratoses – wearing a hat, the use of sun screens, and sun avoidance are all effective.

140 i. The most likely diagnosis is solar urticaria. Differential diagnoses include erythropoietic protoporphyria and polymorphic light eruption.
ii. Many different wavelengths may be responsible and these may belong to the ultraviolet A or B wavebands or even visible wavelengths.
iii. H-1 antihistamines are often helpful in suppressing the weals, but sedation limits their use. Sunscreens may be useful for some patients. Repeated exposure to ultraviolet lamps, fluorescent tubes, or sunlight induces tolerance in many patients and this 'hardening' needs to be repeated on an annual basis. Plasmaphoresis has been successfully employed in patients with a circulating photoallergen.

141 A 73-year-old male presents with a pink but nontender papule that recently appeared on his right cheek and has grown quite rapidly to 1.5 cm in diameter in the previous 3 months. He is quite photodamaged, as a result of his keenness on the outdoor life. He is taking immunosuppressive drugs for rheumatoid arthritis. Biopsy shows that the mass consists of sheets and trabeculae of small cells with dense basophilic nuclei that seem to arise deep in the dermis.
i. Which of the following diagnoses is the most likely and why – pilomatrixoma; epidermoid cyst; Merkel cell tumour; metastatic secondary deposit?
ii. What confirmatory pathology test could be employed for the most likely diagnosis?
iii. What information of pathogenetic interest has recently become available?
iv. What is the recommended treatment and what is the prognosis for the most likely diagnosis?

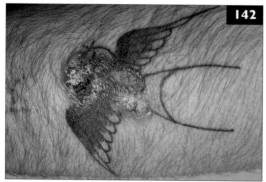

142 i. What is the differential diagnosis of the papules and nodules in this tattoo (**142**)?
ii. What are the dangers of tattooing?
iii. Are there any therapeutic applications of tattooing?

143 A 23-year-old male suddenly develops 'dry scaly' skin. He is also noted to have enlarged lymph nodes in the axillae and neck.
i. What is the likely diagnosis?
ii. What are some other causes of this diagnosis?
iii. Outline the management of this disorder.

141 i. The most likely diagnosis is Merkel cell tumour. This rare neuroendocrine tumour occurs predominantly on the head and neck of elderly white males who are often immunosuppressed. Histologically, it is completely unlike pilomatrixoma or epidermoid cyst, but is often difficult to distinguish from metastatic oat cell carcinoma of the lung.
ii. The presence of cytokeratin 20, as determined immunocytochemically, is regarded as confirmatory.
iii. A specific polyoma virus has been identified in some 80% of cases of Merkel cell tumour.
iv. Early wide excision is the only effective treatment. The tumour metastasizes early and widely (preferentially to lymph nodes). There is an approximate 30% 5-year mortality.

142 i. The differential diagnosis is tattoo granuloma, sarcoidosis, or viral wart.
ii. The main dangers are the blood-borne diseases including human immuno-deficiency virus (HIV) disease, hepatitis B, and syphilis.
iii. Tattoo marks are occasionally made at the site of an intracutaneous test of some sort in order to identify the site. Tattoos with white pigment have been used to camouflage birthmarks or other types of unwanted discolourations.

143 i. The most likely diagnosis is acquired ichthyosis. The generalized persistent scaling but noninflamed condition known as ichthyosis is present at birth and lasts throughout life. When the condition develops in adult life it is known as acquired ichthyosis and is sometimes a sign of an internal malignancy. Hodgkin's disease and the reticuloses are the most common precipitating causes.
ii. Some lipid-lowering agents and the condition of essential fatty acid deficiency may also cause acquired ichthyosis. It has also been described in patients under-going treatment for leprosy.
iii. The management should be directed to treating the underlying disorder. Symptomatic relief may be obtained by the use of frequent applications of emollient creams and lotions and bath preparations.

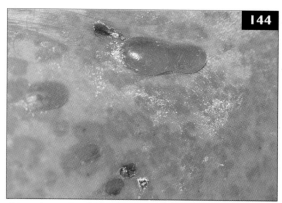

144 A 74-year-old male noticed that his skin felt itchy and that transient red marks developed some weeks before large, tense blood-stained blisters appeared on his arms and legs (144).
i. What is the differential diagnosis?
ii. How will the diagnosis be confirmed?
iii. Discuss the general medical implications of the most likely diagnosis.
iv. Outline the management of this disorder.

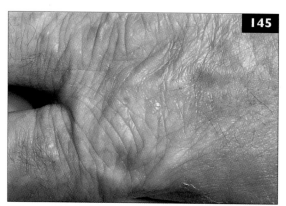

145 A sociable 55-year-old male presents with blisters over the backs of his hands (145) and on the forehead.
i. What is the differential diagnosis?
ii. What physical signs may accompany the most likely diagnosis?
iii. What treatments are available for the most likely diagnosis?

144 i. The most likely diagnosis is senile pemphigoid. The large size and tense walls of the blisters suggest that the blistering is subepidermal. The period before the blisters appeared, marked by pruritus and odd erythematous and eczematous rashes, is also characteristic of pemphigoid. Dermatitis herpetiformis should also be considered but the blisters are much smaller and are grouped at particular sites. The absence of mucosal lesions makes erythema multiforme and pemphigus much less likely. Benign mucosal pemphigoid heals with scarring.
ii. The diagnosis may be confirmed by immunofluorescent tests – for circulating IgG antibodies directed against the subepidermal region (indirect test) and IgG and C3 complement fixed at the dermoepidermal junction of perilesional skin (direct test). A biopsy will confirm that the blistering is subepidermal.
iii. Senile pemphigoid is sometimes a marker of internal malignancy although this is uncommon.
iv. The aim of management is to stop the blistering by employing systemic steroids or immunosuppressive agents.

145 i. A quite likely diagnosis is that of porphyria cutanea tarda (PCT). Blisters in light-exposed sites in middle-aged male subjects who drink alcohol to excess are characteristic. PCT may also occur together with acute intermittent porphyria as an inherited disorder called porphyria variegata. A similar condition can occur after oral furosemide or nalidixic acid – known as 'pseudopophyria'. Blistering can also occur in light-exposed areas as part of a photodermatitis.
ii. Other physical signs include hirsutism, pigmentation, and morphoea-like skin thickening at the affected sites. The diagnosis can be confirmed by estimating the porphyrins in the stools, urine, and blood. In PCT there is an increase in copro-porphyrin III in the stools and urine.
iii. Regular venesection (570 ml [1 pint] per week) controls the disorder. Alternatively, chloroquine by mouth increases porphyrin excretion and controls the disease. Avoidance of sun exposure and use of ultraviolet A-blocking sunscreens helps prevent lesions.

146 A female presents with an increasing number of pinkish papules distributed over the trunk and limbs in the past year (146). They itch and redden when scratched.
i. What is the most likely diagnosis?
ii. What are the systemic components of this disorder?
iii. Outline the management.

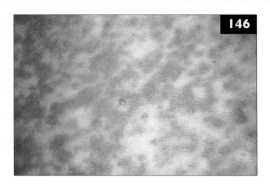

147 The lesions in 147 appeared some 10 days previously and show no signs of remitting. They are tender, red, and swollen. These plaques and papules are confined to the upper arms, face, neck, and upper chest and are accompanied by a remittent fever, malaise, anthralgia, and a polymorphonuclear leucocytosis.
i. What are the most likely diagnosis and differential diagnosis?
ii. Describe the relevant positive laboratory findings.
iii. Could there be a provocative stimulus for the most likely diagnosis?

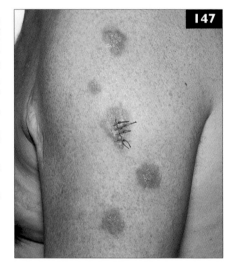

148 A 35-year-old male complains of worsening unpleasant shooting pains, mainly in his limbs but occasionally elsewhere as well. Close examination reveals numerous angiomata over the entire body, which he says have been present for some years. Some of the lesions have a roughened warty surface.
i. What is the differential diagnosis and what is the most likely cause of the problem?
ii. What is the nature of this condition and how is it inherited?
iii. What systemic manifestations develop in this disorder?

146 i. The most likely diagnosis is adult mastocytosis – rubbing or scratching the lesions will often result in redness and sometimes swelling of the area. This is known as Darier's sign and is due to the release of histamine from mast cell granules in the mast cells of the lesion. This may also happen in a hot bath or after administration of some drugs such as opioids.

ii. Mast cell deposits are found in bone, liver, and lungs, but for the most part these abnormalities have no clinical consequence.

iii. It is important to warn affected individuals that they may be subject to attacks of flushing and, if severe enough, fainting. These attacks may be precipitated by alcohol and by drugs, especially morphine alkaloids and curare-like drugs. This is of great importance because if general anaesthesia is induced with drugs that can precipitate these attacks, a serious hypotensive crisis can arise with catastrophic shock and even death.

147 i. The most likely diagnosis is acute neutrophilic dermatosis (Sweet's syndrome). Other possibilities include erythema multiforme, but the lesions are more erosive and there is greater mucosal involvement. Erythema elevatum diutinum is another possibility, but the lesions are more persistent in this condition. Behçet's disease should also be considered.

ii. There are usually a high neutrophil leucocytosis, a high erythrocyte sedimentation rate, and characterisitic skin biopsy findings of a dense dermal infiltrate of numerous neutrophils with neutrophil fragments (leucocytoclasis) and endothelial cell swelling.

iii. Sweet's syndrome is often provoked by underlying disease including leukaemia, myelodysplastic syndromes, inflammatory bowel disease (e.g. Crohn's disease or ulcerative colitis), neoplasms of bowel or breast, and rheumatoid arthritis.

148 i. The skin lesions are angiomata or angiokeratomata and their presence over the whole body together with the symptoms of neuropathic pain are strongly suggestive of angiokeratomata corporis diffusum (Anderson Fabry disease).

ii. This is an uncommon X-linked recessive condition occurring in approximately 1 in 250,000 of the population. It is caused by defective activity of the lysosomal enzyme alpha-galactosidase leading to the deposition of glycosphingolipids (predominantly globotriaosylceramide). These are deposited in lysosomes, particularly those of the cutaneous vascular endothelium.

iii. Because of the widespread deposition of the glycosphingolipds, various organs and systems are affected. Cardiac and renal dysfunction are common, and episodes of severe neuropathic pain and ophthalmic problems are also often present.

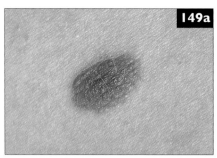

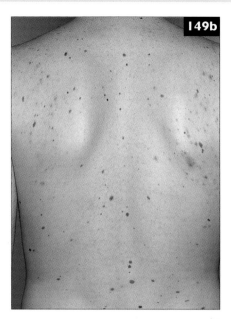

149 A mother is concerned about her son's curious moles, which are odd-looking and numerous (149a, b).
i. What is the condition called and why is the mother worried?
ii. Is there a genetic component to this condition?
iii. How is the disorder best managed?

150 A 67-year-old male is referred by his GP because he is concerned that the painful, tender warty papule on the rim of the external ear is a skin cancer.
i. What is the differential diagnosis and the most likely diagnosis?
ii. What is thought to be the pathogenesis of this disorder?
iii. What treatment is recommended?

151 A boy presents who, since early infancy, cried and screamed shortly after being outside in the sun, although all that could be seen were some red patches, some of them urticarial.
i. What is the diagnosis?
ii. What is the metabolic basis of this disease?
iii. Are there helpful physical signs associated with the condition? To what complications are patients with this disorder subject?

149 i. The condition is known as 'dysplastic mole syndrome'. There are many moles with irregular outlines and variegated pigmentation. There is a much higher likelihood of one of these becoming a malignant melanoma than an ordinary mole. **ii.** Many individuals with this disorder do not have a family history of a similar condition, but a significant proportion do, with the condition being inherited as a Mendelian dominant condition.
iii. All odd moles that have recently enlarged, or changed in shape and colour, should be excised and examined histologically. All other moles should be inspected on a monthly basis by parent/partner. Some dermatologists advocate regular photography so that the growth of any particular mole can be checked objectively.

150 i. The diagnosis is chondrodermatitis nodularis chronica helicis (CDNCH), but solar keratosis or squamous cell carcinoma must also be considered diagnostic possibilities.
ii. Pressure on the ear when sleeping causes ischaemic injury to the area affected.
iii. It should be treated by use of a very soft (e.g. expanded rubber) pillow or by excision of the affected site including the underlying cartilage.

151 i. The disorder has the typical features of erythropoietic protoporphyria.
ii. The disorder is a dominantly inherited condition in which protoporphyrins accumulate in the blood and elsewhere due to defective action of the enzyme ferrochelatase.
iii. Patients develop a characteristic pitted scarring over the bridge of the nose. Some 10% of patients develop pigment gall stones. A few develop serious hepatocellular disease.

152 i. What is the condition illustrated in 152? What is the basis of the disorder?
ii. In what conditions does this disorder occur?
iii. How should this disorder be treated?

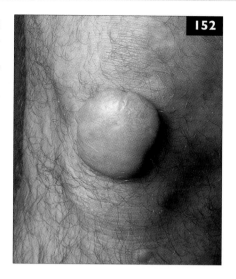

153 The area of skin shown in 153 developed over a 2-week period. It feels firm and has a mauvish hue; the skin seems thickened.
i. What is the most likely diagnosis?
ii. Does the disorder have systemic components? If so, what are these?
iii. Describe the pathology and what is known of the pathogenesis.

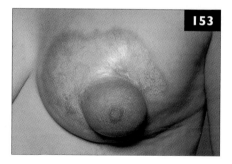

154 i. What are the lesions in 154?
ii. What is the cause of these lesions?
iii. What management should be recommended?

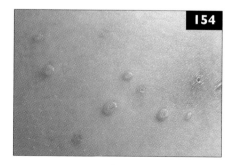

152 i. The condition is xanthoma tuberosum. It is the result of deposition and accumulation of lipid in histiocytes and giant cells throughout the dermis in affected sites.

ii. Xanthoma tuberosum is seen in the condition of essential familial hyper-cholesterolaemia. This condition (type II hyperlipidaemia) is inherited as a dominant characteristic. It is also uncommonly seen in the mixed hyperlipidaemia occurring in diabetes mellitus and in eruptive xanthoma.

iii. Treatment is essentially that of managing the underlying disorder – diet and appropriate blood lipid-lowering drugs.

153 i. The most likely diagnosis is morphoea. A morphoeic basal cell carcinoma may mimic a basal cell carcinoma and areas of scarring may have some features in common with morphoea. Areas of fat atrophy (lipoatrophy) panniculitis may also rarely simulate morphoea.

ii. Morphoea is also known as localized scleroderma, but it is very rare for this localized form to be part of generalized systemic sclerosis. It is also rare (but less rare) for morphoea to spread to involve a wide area of skin (generalized morphoea).

iii. Morphoea is thought to be autoimmune in nature, but the detail of the process is unknown. It is known that new collagen is deposited at the site. A perivascular infiltrate of mononuclear cells is often present, particularly at the periphery of the plaque.

154 i. The condition is molluscum contagiosum. It mainly affects children, especially those with atopic dermatitis, and young adults and is spread by skin-to-skin contact. The umbilicated pearly papules typical of the disorder may be present in large numbers, especially in immunosuppressed individuals.

ii. Molluscum contagiosum is caused by a large DNA virus belonging to the poxvirus group.

iii. The lesions disappear spontaneously within a few months to a year and usually treatment is not required. There is no specific medication available for treatment, but individual lesions can be removed by curettage.

155 A female complains bitterly about the rash on her face, but all that can be seen are a few crusted spots on her chin and some scratch marks (155).
i. What is the most likely diagnosis?
ii. Briefly discuss the pathogenesis.
iii. Discuss the management.

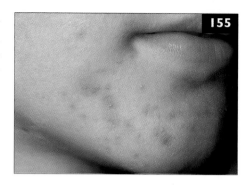

156 A male presents with dark red and mauvish papules and nodules on the legs that are extremely itchy (156). They have been present for 8 months and seem to be enlarging.
i. What is the differential diagnosis?
ii. Describe the typical pathological changes found in the most likely diagnosis.
iii. Outline the management for this disorder.

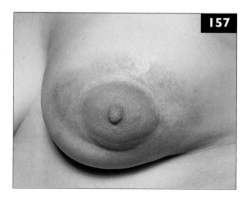

157 A 17-year-old female presents with two thickened areas of skin, one on her back and the other on her breast (157).
i. What is the diagnosis?
ii. Describe the pathology of the disorder.
iii. What is known of the aetiology and pathogenesis of this condition?

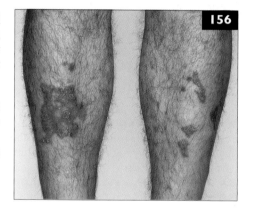

155 i. The most likely diagnosis is '*acne excoriée des jeunes filles*'. This disorder is no more than extensively excoriated minor acne in young women.
ii. It is commonplace for acne patients of both sexes to squeeze, pick or scratch a few of their acne spots. However, in this condition the manual interference is very marked and the patient denies interfering with the lesions. In some instances there is very little acne (if any) but considerable excoriation and the condition is really a type of dermatitis artefacta.
iii. The management is difficult as the urge to try to rid the skin of the offending blemishes is extremely strong. Topical treatment for the acne should be prescribed as well as discussion concerning the need to stop interfering with the lesions.

156 i. The most likely diagnosis is hypertrophic lichen planus. Other possibilities include prurigo nodularis and lymphoma. The diagnosis would be assisted by finding typical lichen planus papules elsewhere or lichen planus lesions affecting the buccal mucosa.
ii. The typical histological picture shows marked epidermal thickening, amounting to pseudoepitheliomatous hyperplasia in some cases. The characteristic histo-pathology of lichen planus with basal cell erosion, cytoid body formation, and sawtooth profile architecture may not be prominent, but is usually present some-where in the sample. Other features, such as the hypergranulosis and hyper-keratosis, as well as the subepidermal mononuclear 'lichenoid' band, are variably present.
iii. Lesions of hypertrophic lichen planus may persist for several years if untreated. Potent topical corticosteroids may give some relief. Other treatments that may assist include topical tacrolimus and systemic ciclosporin.

157 i. The diagnosis is localized scleroderma (morphoea). The differential diagnosis includes scars and scleroderma-like change seen in porphyria cutanea tarda.
ii. Histologically, the dermis is thickened because of its content of featureless pale-staining bundles of collagen in the deep dermis. In new lesions there is also a perivascular lymphocytic cellular infiltrate.
iii. It is thought that morphoea is closely related to systemic sclerosis, which is part of the autoimmune spectrum of diseases.

158 A 52-year-old female presents with a red nodule (1.5 cm²) on her right upper thigh that has been unchanging for the last 15 years (158a). It is red, has a glazed shiny surface, but causes no discomfort.
i. What is the most likely diagnosis?
ii. Describe the pathology of this condition.
iii. What is the prognosis if untreated? What is the recommended treatment?

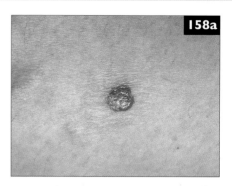

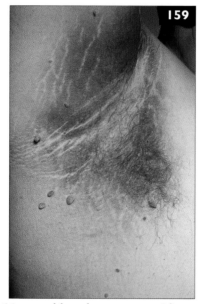

159 An overweight 66-year-old male presents with numerous skin tags and pigmented seborrhoeic warts in the axillae (159), at the sides of his neck, and in the groins.
i. What is this condition?
ii. From what disorder must it be distinguished?
iii. What is known about its pathogenesis?

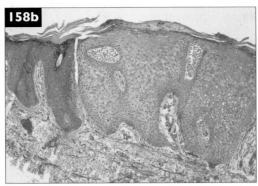

158 i. The clinical description fits the condition known as 'clear cell acanthoma' (Degos acanthoma). Characteristically, these benign lesions have a glazed red appearance and are present unchanging for many years.

ii. Figure **158b** shows the main pathological features of this condition. Note that it consists of an irregularly thickened epidermis containing large pale (glycogen-laden) epidermal cells, save in the basal layers, which consist of small basophilic cells. The epidermis is invaded by polymorphonuclear leucocytes and overall the picture is somewhat reminiscent of plaque-type psoriasis.

iii. If untreated, the lesions persist. The most appropriate treatment is surgical excision.

159 i. The patient is suffering from the condition known as pseudoacanthosis nigricans. This condition, which is characterized by hyperpigmentation and increased rugosity of the skin of the major flexures, is also marked by the development of numerous filiform and warty papillomatous skin tag lesions and an increase in number, size, and pigmentation of seborrhoeic warts. It is almost identical with true acanthosis nigricans, but is not associated with underlying endocrine or malignant disease; it is positively associated with obesity.

ii. It must be distinguished from true acanthosis nigricans. In the latter condition there are also changes in the buccal mucosa and on the palms. True acanthosis nigricans is associated either with endocrine disease or with an underlying visceral malignancy.

iii. Not very much is known about the pathogenesis other than these patients are mostly diabetic and demonstrate a high level of insulin resistance.

160 A 57-year-old male presents with a brown patch beneath the right great toe nail, which first appeared 4 months previously and seems to be increasing in size (**160**).
i. What is the differential diagnosis?
ii. Briefly discuss the management.
iii. Briefly discuss the incidence and prognosis of the most serious of the diagnostic possibilities.

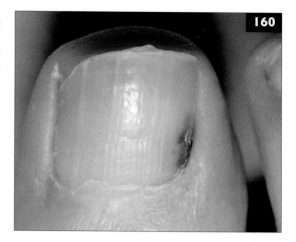

161 An elderly male presents because his skin seems to have become drier and itchier; no other abnormality can be found on his skin or elsewhere.
i. What is the diagnosis?
ii. What are the main points in his management?
iii. Briefly comment on the cause and prognosis.

162 i. What is the lesion seen in **162**?
ii. What is the explanation for its presence?
iii. What other lesions may accompany the condition illustrated?

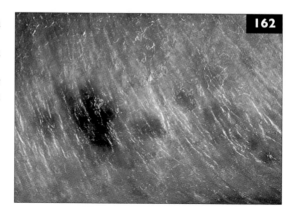

160 i. A benign naevus can uncommonly appear late in life. The commonest cause for the subungual pigmentation is a haematoma. The major concern is whether the lesion is a subungual melanoma or not. Unfortunately this diagnosis can be very difficult to distinguish from a haematoma. A fungal infection can cause a brown–black discolouration, but the nail plate is usually affected.
ii. If there is any doubt at all that the lesion could be a melanoma, the nail should be removed and a biopsy of the lesion performed.
iii. Subungal melanoma is a form of acral lentiginous melanoma, which is more frequent in Asian and African peoples, but uncommon in the west. The overall prognosis is worse than for other forms of melanoma.

161 i. This condition is termed senile pruritus. Before making the diagnosis it is essesntial to ensure that there are no other causes for generalized itching, such as systemic disease or scabies.
ii. Care must be taken to ensure that the skin is adequately hydrated by the use of emollients (topically applied and during bathing). Bathing should be in lukewarm water with patting dry and application of emollients afterwards. Clothing should be light and smooth.
iii. The cause of this common distressing condition is unknown. The condition is persistent, but fluctuates in severity, tending to worsen in winter.

162 i. The crimson macules on the backs of the forearms are characteristic of the condition known as senile purpura. A better term would be solar purpura as they appear to be associated with chronic solar damage rather than old age.
ii. The lesions appear in areas of severe chronic solar damage ('photodamage'). They are probably the result of minor injury to the vasculature, which is un-protected because of the replacement of dermal collagen by mechanically inefficient solar elastotic tissue.
iii. Other lesions seen in areas of photodamage are senile lentigines, solar keratoses, basal cell carcinoma, lesions of Bowen's disease, and squamous cell carcinoma. In addition, solar elastotic degenerative change may give rise to a sallow yellowish background colour and permit wrinkles to develop.

163 A male presents with a rash on his ankles and lower legs. It does not itch and seems to be slowly increasing in extent. It consists of red dots and brown spots (163). The full blood picture is normal. The Hess test is negative.
i. What is the most likely diagnosis and what is the differential diagnosis?
ii. What are the pathogenesis and pathology of the most likely diagnosis?
iii. Briefly discuss the management of this disorder.

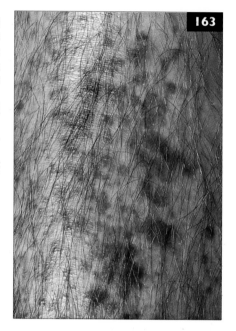

164 A 45-year-old female complains of pain and coldness of the right lower leg that has gradually become worse over the previous 3 weeks. On examination the peripheral pulses are absent, the right lower leg is cold to the touch, and there is incipient necrosis of the right big toe. The patient admits to smoking three cannabis cigarettes per day.
i. What is the diagnosis and what is the main differential diagnosis?
ii. How common is this condition?
iii. What treatment is recommended and what is the prognosis?

165 A male presents with myriads of filiform warts covering the sides of his neck. They have been present for at least 5 years.
i. What are the possible explanations for ths eruption of warts?
ii. What other skin infections may act in this way?
iii. How should the condition be managed?

163 i. The presence of red dots and brown spots strongly suggests that the condition is a form of capillaritis. As there is no thrombocytopenia or systematic capillaropathy, the condition is likely to be one of the capillaritis group. The most frequent of those, occurring predominantly on the legs of young men, is Schamberg's disease. The differential diagnosis includes thrombocytopenic purpura and drug-induced purpura as well as bacteraemic conditions such as subacute bacterial endocarditis, gonococcaemia, and meningococcaemia.
ii. The pathology is undramatic. The papillary dermis is the main site of abnormality. Characteristically, there is extravasated blood and some blood pigment around the papillary capillaries as well as a few inflammatory cells. Nothing is known of the cause of the disorder.
iii. The diagnosis needs to be established by the appropriate tests. The condition is asymptomatic and eventually fades. No treatment is required.

164 i. The diagnosis is cannabis arteritis. The main differential diagnosis is thromboangiitis obliterans which can closely resemble cannabis arteritis, although as this patient is female thrombangitis is most unlikely.
ii. Cannabis arteritis is not very common, but is an occasional problem.
iii. Patients must stop smoking cannabis as well as stopping smoking ordinary cigarettes. At the same time they should be given aspirin (75–100 mg daily). Infusions of the prostaglandin analogue iloprost may also be given. If the patient complies and the disease is treated before there has been much tissue necrosis, the outlook is excellent and limbs and digits are usually saved.

165 i. The usual explanation for the rare occurrence of myriads of warts is some form of immunosuppression, such as occurs in human immunodeficiency virus (HIV) disease, or accompanies Hodgkin's disease or other lymphoma, or a congenital immunodeficiency. However, occasionally no underlying immunodeficiency is found.
ii. Molluscum contagiosum, pityriasis versicolor, and herpes simplex are amongst other skin infections that may be widespread due to underlying immunodeficiency.
iii. Any underlying immunodeficiency needs to be identified and if possible treated. Appropriate topical treatment with virucidal agents or keratolytic agents may be offered after treatment of the immune deficit.

166 This patient began to develop smooth pink nodules on her scalp at the age of 23 and more have gradually appeared in the intervening years (166).
i. What is this condition? How can the diagnosis be confirmed?
ii. Is there a strong possibility of a family history of this disorder?
iii. What complications are well known to occur?
iv. What management would be recommended?

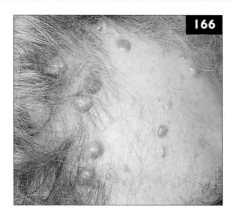

167 **i.** The woman in 167 is only 55 years old. Why does she look so very much older?
ii. Wrinkling is the characteristic feature of the condition from which she suffers – what is the main histological feature? What else can have the same effect?
iii. What other clinical signs are often found in this condition?

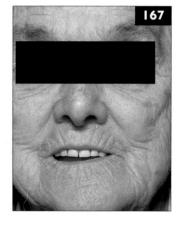

168 The lesion whose pathology is illustrated (168) felt quite hard to the touch before it was removed.
i. What is the diagnosis?
ii. Explain and describe the typical histological features.
iii. In whom does the lesion usually occur and at what anatomical sites?

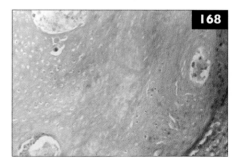

166 i. This patient has the typical features of cylindroma. Histological examination of an excised lesion will show a characteristic picture of large nodules of basaloid cells within the dermis containing some larger cells and surrounded by a pink hyaline featureless band.
ii. The condition is inherited in a Mendelian dominant fashion, but is mainly seen in women.
iii. The condition is a hamartomatous benign naevoid disorder and not subject to any serious complications.
iv. Affected individuals may possess large numbers of these benign tumours and unfortunately it is just not feasible to remove many of these. Most patients appear to accept their presence with equanimity.

167 i. The woman suffers from photodamage due to chronic excessive exposure to the sun's ultraviolet radiation.
ii. The main histological feature is an alteration in the dermal connective tissue known as solar elastotic degenerative change (solar elastosis), in which the usual dermal fibrous arrangement gives way to a disorganized basophilic structure consisting of globular homogeneous areas and short wavy strands. Chronic heat injury, radiotherapy, and smoking are other causes of 'elastosis'.
iii. Solar keratoses, areas of dyspigmentation, and telangiectasia and ecchymoses are other features of photodamage.

168 i. The lesion is a pilomatrixoma (also known as calcifying epithelioma of Malherbe).
ii. At the periphery are basaloid epithelial cells. These degenerate into 'ghost cells', which later calcify. Contact with surrounding tissues results in granulomatous inflammation with prominent giant cell systems.
iii. These lesions often occur in adolescents and young adults and are for the most part on the head or neck or upper limbs.

169 A 55-year-old male complains of a sore mouth and some moist eroded or blistered patches on the skin of the chest and back (169) during the previous 3 weeks. They have not responded to any topical medication used and new lesions have continued to appear. A biopsy is reported as showing a suprabasilar split and acantholysis.
i. What is the most likely diagnosis?
ii. What immunological findings might be present?
iii. Outline the management of this disease.

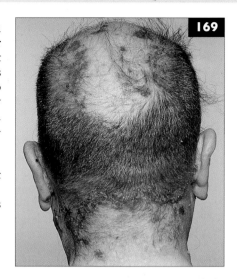

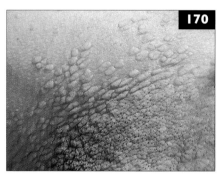

170 A male presents with a large number of small whitish papules around his mouth and nose (170). They have been present for the past 6 weeks and have been increasing in number.
i. What is the most likely diagnosis?
ii. What is the cause of these lesions?
iii. Discuss the treatment for this condition.

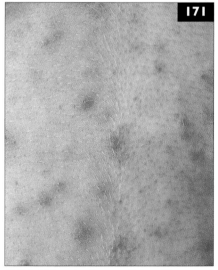

171 i. What is the condition illustrated in 171?
ii. What are the main clinical features?
iii. How is it inherited?
iv. What are the main complications?

169 i. The most likely diagnosis is pemphigus vulgaris, although lichen planus and fixed drug eruption are other possibilities.
ii. In this serious blistering autoimmune disorder there are circulating complement fixing antibodies to proteins of the desmosomal complex of the epidermis. The localization of these antibodies can be demonstrated in the indirect immuno-fluorescence test on skin taken from near the lesions.
iii. The disease can be suppressed by large doses of oral steroids and an immuno-suppressant drug such as ciclosporin, azathioprine, or methotrexate. Systemic gold therapy has also been used successfully. In recent years biological agents such as rituximab and infliximab have been reported to be effective treatments.

170 i. The most likely diagnosis is plane warts. They are sometimes confused with small acne spots or the lesions of mollusca contagiosa.
ii. Plane warts are caused by human papillomavirus of antigenic type 5. They may well have been implanted and spread by shaving. Outbreaks tend to be more frequent and more extensive in immunosuppressed individuals.
iii. Where there are only a few lesions one option is to offer no treatment, as they often remit after a few weeks. Alternatively, they can be destroyed by cautery and curettage or by cryotherapy. Topical agents containing salicylic acid are also useful over limited areas.

171 i. The condition illustrated is neurofibromatosis (type 1), or Von Reckling-hausen's disease.
ii. The main clinical features are the presence of multiple soft, pink or skin-coloured nodules over the trunk, which histologically are neurofibromata and brown macules (*café au lait* patches).
iii. The condition is inherited as an autosomal dominant condition, although 50% of cases are the result of new mutations.
iv. Neural tumours, including gliomata and meningiomata, are said to occur more commonly. Leiomyomas (including cardiac leiomyomas) are more common, as are phaeochromocytomas.

172 A 9-month-old boy presents with a red mark over the left side of his face and neck (172).

i. What is this lesion and what is the prognosis?

ii. What disability does it cause and what is the pathological picture of this lesion?

iii. What treatments may be recommended?

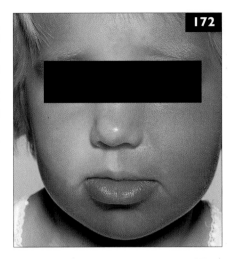

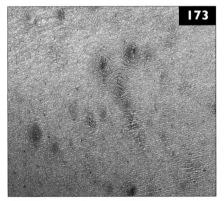

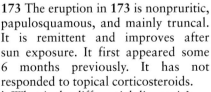

173 The eruption in 173 is nonpruritic, papulosquamous, and mainly truncal. It is remittent and improves after sun exposure. It first appeared some 6 months previously. It has not responded to topical corticosteroids.

i. What is the differential diagnosis?

ii. Are there characteristic features of the most likely diagnosis?

iii. Discuss the management of this patient.

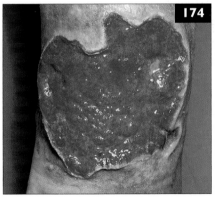

174 A 47-year-old male, who has not enjoyed good health in recent years, presents with a large inflamed lump on the side of his lower leg which, after 2 weeks, becomes a large spreading ulcer (174).

i. What is the most likely diagnosis?

ii. What underlying disorders are associated with this condition?

iii. Decribe appropriate management for this condition.

172 i. This is a port wine stain. On the face it is often in the distribution of one of the branches of the trigeminal nerve. Unlike some congenital vascular malformations, it does not improve with time: if anything it tends to thicken and become more prominent in middle age.
ii. Port wine stains often cause very serious disability because of the cosmetic deformity resulting in immense psychological disturbance.
iii. When cosmetic disability is minimal, cosmetic camouflage may suffice. Many patients do well with a course of laser treatment with pulsed dye laser at an age when the child can cooperate. The treatment needs to be designed and administered by a laser expert.

173 i. The possible diagnoses include psoriasis, mycosis fungoides, and pityriasis lichenoides chronica, which is the most likely diagnosis.
ii. The dermatopathological picture typically shows the presence of a detaching parakeratotic scale, infiltration of the epidermis by mononuclear cells, sparse scattered degenerate keratinocytes, and a subepidermal mononuclear inflammatory cell infiltrate.
iii. No pharmacological interventions seem to produce significant improvement, but treatment by ultraviolet B radiation does seem to produce a temporary remission.

174 i. The condition is pyoderma gangrenosum. Characteristically, it starts as an inflamed nodule, which then breaks down into a rapidly spreading ulcer. The ulcer edge is slightly raised, bluish, and undermined.
ii. Pyoderma gangrenosum is associated with a number of systemic disorders including ulcerative colitis, rheumatoid arthritis, and multiple myeloma. It can also occur spontaneously without a detectable underlying disease.
iii. Apart from supportive and antimicrobial treatment, good results have been reported for ciclosporin, tacrolimus, doxycycline, dapsone, and infliximab.

175 A female infant presents with itchy red bumps that appeared in the past few weeks. They come in waves and are quite troublesome. The spots seem to last for 2–3 days before fading and leaving a bruise-like stain (175).
i. What is the diagnosis?
ii. How can the diagnosis be confirmed?
iii. Discuss the management.

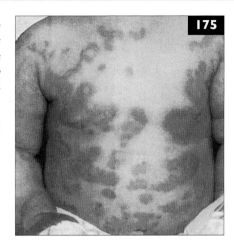

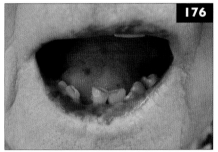

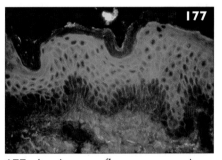

176 A female presents with pigmented patches on her lips (176). She also has pigmented areas on the buccal mucosa and over the backs of the fingers and scattered pigmented macules elsewhere. In addition, she has had bouts of abdominal pain, one of which was accompanied by melaena. She reports that her father and a brother also have the same problem.
i. What is the diagnosis?
ii. Briefly comment on the aetiopathogenesis.
iii. What are the complications of this disorder?

177 An immunofluorescence microphotograph using anti-human immunoglobulin G (IgG) serum linked to fluorescein isothiocyanate is shown (177).
i. What is the diagnosis?
ii. What other blistering disorders have an immunopathogenesis?
iii. What skin disorders are marked by deposits of IgG at the dermoepidermal junction?

175 i. The diagnosis is most likely urticarial vasculitis. Other possible diagnoses include ordinary urticaria and insect bites.

ii. The diagnosis can be confirmed by biopsy; the histological appearance is distinctive, with swelling of the capillary endothelium and fragmented polymorphonuclear leucocytes.

iii. Urticarial vasculitis may be seen in the course of lupus erythematosus and dermatitis herpetiformis. It may also be part of the picture of a systemic vasculitis. In these cases the management is that of the underlying diseases. Antihistamines are ineffectual. To control the appearance of new lesions, systemic steroids or immunosuppressive drugs should be used.

176 i. The diagnosis is Peutz–Jeghers (P–J) syndrome.

ii. P–J syndrome is a rare congenital disorder which is inherited in an autosomal dominant fashion.

iii. In P–J syndrome polyps characteristically occur anywhere in the gastrointestinal tract. Symptoms from these are common and due to intussusception or bleeding causing anaemia. Furthermore, as the patient ages there is an increasing chance of malignant changes in the polyps. It should be noted that malignant disease from viscera other than the gastrointestinal tract are also more frequent.

177 i. The diagnosis is that of pemphigus vulgaris. IgG and C3 are deposited in the intercellular areas and are thought to be responsible for the acantholysis.

ii. Senile pemphigoid, in which large subepidermal blisters form, dermatitis herpetiformis, in which small subepidermal itchy blisters form, and pemphigoid gestationis, in which itchy subepidermal blisters form in pregnant women, are some other important blistering disorders with an immunopathogenesis; however, there are many others.

iii. Lupus erythematosus and lichen planus are other skin disorders in which IgG is deposited at the dermoepidermal junction.

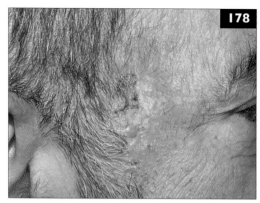

178 A male presents with lesions on his head (178) that first appeared about 10 months previously. They are sore and moist at times, they seem to always appear at the same sites, and they seem subject to spontaneous remission and relapse. There is some evidence of scarring at the affected sites.
i. What is the most likely diagnosis?
ii. What investigations will assist with diagnosis?
iii. Discuss the prognosis and management.

179 i. What is the condition seen in 179?
ii. Who develop this condition?
iii. What is it due to?

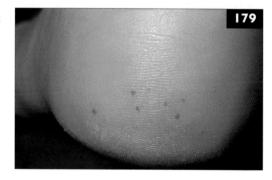

180 A male developed tense blisters on the legs that have healed with scarring. He has a long history of Crohn's disease.
i. What is the most likely clinical diagnosis?
ii. Outline the pathology and pathogenesis of this disease.
iii. Comment on the inter-relationships with other blistering diseases.

178 i. The most likely diagnosis is cicatricial pemphigoid (chronic benign mucous membrane pemphigoid). This disorder has the characteristic of reappearing at the same sites on the skin and/or mucosae. It is mainly a disorder of elderly subjects. Pemphigus foliaceous should also be considered, but this disorder tends to spread and does not have the same tendency to heal with scars.

ii. A biopsy may or may not confirm that the disorder is characterized by sub-epidermal blistering, depending on where the biopsy is taken from. There is often a marked inflammatory cell infiltrate in the upper dermis and there may be evidence of scar formation. Immunofluorescence studies do not show a consistent pattern either of circulating antibodies or immunoprotein deposits in affected skin.

iii. Cicatricial pemphigoid is a persistent disorder characterized by repeated sudden bouts of disease activity. The affected sites show gradual increases in scarring and this may be a major problem for patients with mucosal lesions. These latter are not uncommon in the conjunctivae and this can lead to a serious problem because of the formation of adhesions (synechiae) with impairment of visual function. Buccal mucosal lesions may also be troublesome. Lesions may be treated with potent topical corticosteroids; in severely affected patients systemic steroids or immuno-modulating agents may be used.

179 i. The condition is known as 'talon noir' or black heel disease.
ii. It is seen in squash players.
iii. It is thought to be due to the shearing forces experienced by the heels during the rapid turning movements in the game of squash causing rupture of the eccrine sweat ducts and their filling up with blood.

180 i. The most likely clinical diagnosis is epidermolyis bullosa acquisita (EBA). The condition is characterized by spontaneous blistering as well as blistering after trauma, healing with scarring, and formation of milia and erosions – clinical features quite like those of dystrophic epidermolyis bullosa (EB). Inflammatory bowel disease is a common precursor of EBA.

ii. The blistering is subepidermal and the site of damage is in the collagen VII of the anchoring fibrils of the lamina densa. Antibodies to this region and fixation of antibodies at this site can be detected.

iii. This condition was called EBA because clinically it has some similarities to dystrophic EB, in which there is an inherited problem of anchoring fibril synthesis. There is also some resemblance to bullous lupus erythematosus and cicatricial pemphigoid.

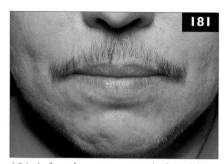

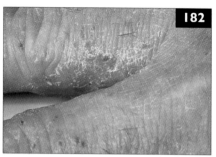

181 A female presents with facial hair that first became a cosmetic problem for her at the age of 27 (181). Hair sprouted from the chin and she has developed a moustache. There is also increased hair on the arms and legs and some on the chest.
i. What are the main possible causes of her hirsutism?
ii. What physical signs indicate the presence of a virilization syndrome?
iii. What are the main methods for removing facial hair?

182 A male presents with an irritating rash on his hands that began 3 months ago and slowly spread (182). He works in an electronics factory.
i. What is the most likely diagnosis?
ii. What are the probable effects of the condition for the patient?
iii. Outline the management of this case.

183 A female presents with a pink–red rash, composed of micropapules, which runs in a linear fashion all the way down the back of her leg (183). It has been there for 2 months and shows no sign of shifting.
i. What is this disorder?
ii. What other diagnoses need be considered?
iii. Who typically suffer from the condition?
iv. What is the management and what is the prognosis of this disorder?

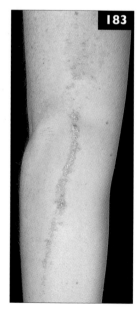

181 i. The main causes are 'idiopathic', ethnic or familial, polycystic ovarian syndrome, androgen-secreting tumour, and administration of anabolic steroids and ciclosporin.

ii. The presence of acne, 'greasy skin', the development of male pattern alopecia, increase in musculature.

iii. Shaving (unpopular!), the use of chemical depilatories (thioglycollates), 'wax' removal, electrical epilation (electrolysis) and, most recently, laser hair removal.

182 i. The most likely diagnosis is chronic primary irritant dermatitis. Allergic contact dermatitis is likely to have a different distribution dependent on the allergen. Psoriasis can be difficult to distinguish but tends to be more circumscribed and less irritating.

ii. The patient may be disturbed over the appearance of his rash as it is unattractive. It may limit his hand movements because his hands will be stiffer and the skin tends to crack when stretched. The irritation is likely to be disturbing.

iii. The cause of his rash needs identification and he needs to be patch tested to exclude the possibility of allergic contact dermatitis. Initially he ought to have a period away from any type of manual work. Emollients will be required as will weak corticosteroids.

183 i. The pink micropapules (1–3 mm diameter) arranged along Blaschko lines in 1–3 cm bands are quite typically due to lichen striatus.

ii. The differential diagnoses include linear lichen planus, linear psoriasis, and epidermal naevus.

iii. Typically, the condition affects females aged 3–12 years. It is not uncommon for siblings to also be affected and it has been noted that the condition occurs more often in the summer months.

iv. The condition resolves spontaneously within 1 year in most cases and treatment is not needed.

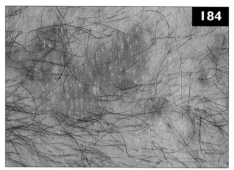

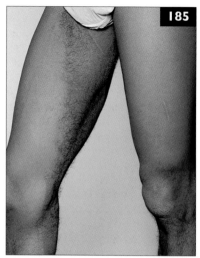

184 This plaque-like lesion (**184**) has been slowly growing over the abdomen in the previous 2 years.
i. What is the likely diagnosis? Are there other diagnoses that should be considered?
ii. Discuss the pathology of the likely diagnosis.
iii. Discuss the management of this condition.

185 A 21-year-old male presents with an area of thickened skin that first affected his left thigh when he was 13 or 14 years of age. It has gradually become darker and more hairy (**185**).
i. What is the likely explanation for this patient's skin disorder?
ii. Describe the pathology of the most likely diagnosis.
iii. Briefly discuss the management.

186 A 12-year-old female presents with an itchy sore rash on both forefeet, worse on the left, which has been present for the past 3 months. It has a 'glazed' red appearance and the skin is scaling and fissured in places (**186**).
i. What is the differential diagnosis and which of these is the most likely?
ii. What is known of the cause of the most likely diagnosis?
iii. Discuss the treatment and prognosis.

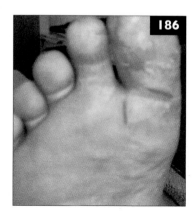

184 i. Dermatofibrosarcoma protuberans is the most likely diagnosis. In the differential diagnosis one should include scar (keloid scar in particular), sclerosing basal cell carcinoma, and other rare connective tissue tumours such as dermato-myofibroma.
ii. The histological picture is not unlike a dermatofibroma, although it is more monomorphic consisting mainly of swirls of spindle-shaped cells often in a 'storiform' arrangement. There is a tendency for there to be a 'cartwheel' pattern in places.
iii. The lesion must be excised with a generous margin to prevent recurrence. Care must be taken at its inferior margins as it tends to infiltrate deeper structures. The prognosis is good, although metastasis does rarely occur.

185 i. This disorder is almost certainly Becker's naevus. This is a congenital disorder that usually affects part of one of the limb girdles. It becomes evident at puberty, gradually becoming more prominent over the next decade. These lesions are essentially epidermal naevi and contain no naevus cells. Amongst other possible diagnoses are the giant naevus cell naevus and naevus of Ota type lesions.
ii. All elements of the epidermal structure show hypertrophy. The epidermis is thickened and there is an increased number of melanocytes in the basal layer. The hair follicles are also increased in number and size.
iii. Unfortunately, not a great deal can be done to improve the appearance. Heroic attempts to excise and graft can lead to disasters and should be resisted. Attempts at reducing the prominence and depth of colour using lasers have as yet been unsuccessful.

186 i. The most likely diagnosis is juvenile plantar dermatosis (JPD), which seems a specific type of eczema, but other red and scaling skin conditions, such as psoriasis and ringworm, need to be considered.
ii. Very little is known of the cause of JPD but it has been suspected that some recent innovation in footwear for the young is to blame (e.g. trainers [sneakers]). Children aged 1–17 years of age are affected and more girls than boys develop the condition.
iii. The prognosis is good as all patients eventually recover. The condition responds slowly (if at all) to topical corticosteroids and more traditional topical medications.

187 A patient with trisomy 21 presents because he has developed odd papular lesions in a serpiginous pattern on the upper trunk and the back of the neck (187) over the past few weeks.
i. What is the diagnosis?
ii. What are the typical histological features?
iii. Name other examples of the process involved.

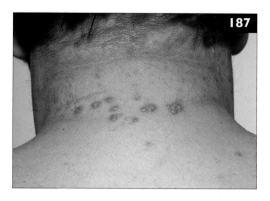

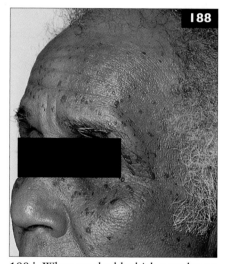

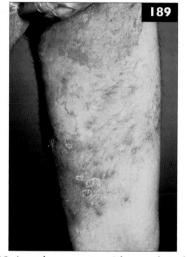

188 i. What are the blackish papules on this patient's face (188)?
ii. What is their significance?
iii. Describe their histological appearance.

189 A male presents with a rash in his groin that is very itchy and has spread very quickly (189). He has been given several topical corticosteroids, but these only seem to encourage the spread of the rash.
i. What is the most likely diagnosis?
ii. What investigations should be performed?
iii. Outline the management.

187 i. The diagnosis is elastosis perforans serpiginosa (EPS) one of the 'perforating disorders' in which dead or damaged dermal material is expelled to the exterior in the process of transepidermal elimination. EPS occurs as an associated disorder in trisomy 21.

ii. Clumps of basophilic elastotic material can be seen in the upper dermis, some in the process of expulsion in distorted and dilated hair follicles. The epidermis shows irregular thickening.

iii. Other disorders in which 'perforation' is seen include perforating collagenoma, necrobiosis lipoidica, and chondrodermatitis nodularis chronica helicis.

188 i. These lesions are known as dermatosis papulosa nigra and are thought to be the equivalent of seborrhoeic warts in black-skinned individuals.

ii. They are benign and have no particular significance other than being associated with ageing.

iii. They have an identical appearance to ordinary seborrhoeic warts except that they contain more pigment.

189 i. The diagnosis is almost certainly 'tinea incognito' or steroid-aggravated ringworm.

ii. The most important investigation is microscopy and culture of skin scrapings; often, large amounts of ringworm fungus can be recovered.

iii. Care must be taken to ensure that no further topical corticosteroids are used. An oral antifungal agent such as terbinafine should be given (250 mg daily) for 1 month and a topical antifungal agent such as miconazole cream should also be prescribed.

190 A child was referred to the paediatrician because he had a series of epileptic seizures. He is referred to the dermatologist because of his facial lesions (190).
i. What is the probable diagnosis?
ii. What other physical signs should be looked for to confirm the suspected condition?
iii. What is the histology of the facial lesions in the suspected condition?

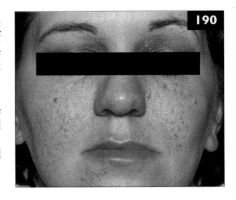

191 A female has had numerous excoriated itchy pink or red nodules on her arms, legs, and trunk for the past 9 months (191). The itch has been disabling and nothing seems to help.
i. What is the most likely diagnosis?
ii. Describe the main histopathological features.
iii. Briefly discuss the management of this condition.

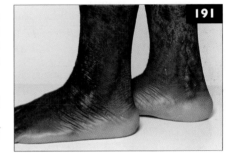

192 A 23-year-old male presents with small, rounded, skin-coloured, cystic papules that have appeared mainly over the upper trunk, but also on the arms, head, and neck in the past 6 months (192). His sister and father also have similar lesions.
i. What is the most likely diagnosis?
ii. What is known of the aetiopathogenesis of this disorder?
iii. Describe the pathology of the condition.

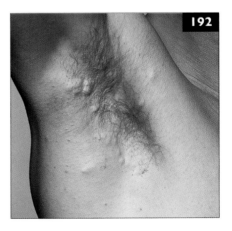

190 i. The probable diagnosis is adenoma sebaceum (tuberous sclerosis). This is a congenital multisystem disorder in which intracerebral fibrotic nodules form, causing an epileptic focus.

ii. Apart from the facial papules, other recorded cutaneous features include white leaf-like patches over the trunk and small fibrous nodules are found around the finger and toe nails (periungal fibromata).

iii. The papular lesions may look acneiform clinically, but histologically they consist of clusters of small blood vessels and fibrous tissue (angiofibromata).

191 i. The condition is known as nodular prurigo. Very little is known of the initiating cause of this condition.

ii. The main histological features are those of massive focal epidermal thickening, more marked than in lichen simplex chronicus. The epidermal thickening may be dramatic and in some instances can qualify for the term 'pseudoepitheliomatous hyperplasia'.

iii. Management is difficult as topical medication (even potent topical corticosteroids) rarely helps. Oral thalidomide may help, but has to be given in low doses and with extreme caution to avoid both the teratogenic and neuropathic adverse side-effects.

192 i. The most likely diagnosis is that of sebocystoma (or steatocystoma) multiplex.

ii. The condition appears to arise from the pilosebaceous structures for unknown reasons. It may be inherited as a dominant characteristic.

iii. Histologically, it can be seen that the lesions are essentially cysts whose walls are often a single layer of nonkeratinizing cuboidal cells, but may also consist of a squamous epithelium. The cyst walls may also contain sebaceous glands and the cyst may contain pure sebum.

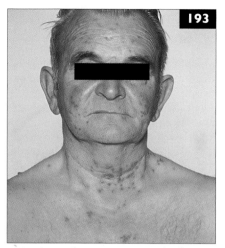

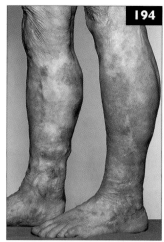

193 A male presents with lesions scattered over his upper trunk and his face. They are dull red or brownish in colour and very persistent (193).
i. What is the diagnosis?
ii. What features would be expected in a biopsy?
iii. Briefly outline the prognosis and management.

194 A 49-year-old male presents with a nonpruritic rash on his lower legs (194). It started some 6 weeks before he attended the clinic and is gradually becoming more prominent. Examination reveals areas of brown pigmentation, some purpuric spots, many dilated venules, and some ankle swelling.
i. What is the diagnosis? What physical signs support the diagnosis?
ii. What histopathological features might one expect to find in a biopsy?
iii. What is the prognosis and how should the patient be managed?

195 A 72-year-old male presents with papules that have appeared on his face (195). They have not increased much in size and are orange–yellow in colour.
i. What is the differential diagnosis? What is the most likely diagnosis?
ii. Describe the histopathological appearance.
iii. What is known of the pathogenesis of the most likely diagnosis?

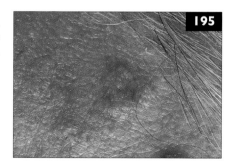

193 i. Acne agminata is the most likely diagnosis. The condition is also known as lupus miliaris disseminatus faciei and as acnitis.
ii. The histological picture usually shows a caseating granuloma with large histiocytes and giant cells surrounding an area of caseation necrosis centrally.
iii. The disorder is self-limiting but takes many months to remit, leaving a pock scar when it does. There is no effective treatment.

194 i. The diagnosis is 'venous hypertension'. The pigmentation, the prominent dilated venules, the petechial spots, and the ankle swelling all support this diagnosis.
ii. Histologically, the capillaries seem increased in number and to be thickened. Some seem to have a fibrin ring around them. Scattered around and between the vessels there is a mixture of inflammatory cells, extravasated red cells, and particles of pigment.
iii. All measures to improve venous drainage should be adopted, including leg elevation on a regular daily basis, support stockings or bandaging, weight reduction, and gentle exercise.

195 i. The differential diagnosis includes senile sebaceous gland hyperplasia (SSGH), basal cell carcinoma, and nonpigmented dermal cellular naevus. The most likely diagnosis is SSGH.
ii. The histological picture characteristically shows lobules of enlarged hyperplastic sebaceous gland tissue quite near the skin surface.
iii. Little is known of the pathogenesis of SSGH, although it does appear to be associated with photodamage in some patients.

196 A 3-year-old boy has complained repeatedly that he has a 'sore bottom'. The perianal region has a few raised areas (196).
i. What is the most likely diagnosis?
ii. What are these lesions caused by?
iii. What should the careful doctor be on the lookout for?

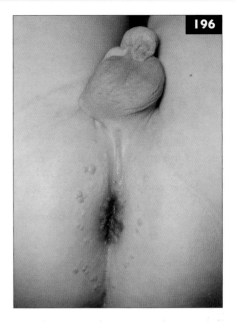

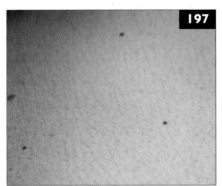

197 A 68-year-old male presents with bright red, dome-shaped lesions over his abdomen (197) each about 3 mm in diameter. There are several other similar lesions over his trunk, which he has not noticed.
i. What are these lesions?
ii. What is their significance for the general health of the individual and what is their natural history?
iii. Describe their histopathological features.

196 i. The perianal soreness was due to the crop of perianal warts. They are usually multiple and around the anal ring. They are usually a shade of pink or creamy white, have warty fronds and sometimes plaques.
ii. These perianal warts are examples of infection by the human papillomavirus of several antigenic types including 16 and 18.
iii. Perianal warts are sometimes the sign of sexual abuse. Other signs should be looked for such as bruising and scratch marks.

197 i. These are typical Campbell de Morgan spots or senile angiomas. They are usually multiple, appearing at about the age of 60 years or later.
ii. They have no significance for the general health. They tend to gradually increase in number and to persist.
iii. Histologically, they consist of proliferated endothelial cells and vascular channels, very similar to the changes in strawberry angioma.

Index

157

Index

Index

Index